FLUID THERAPY
in dogs and cats

Fabio Viganò
Deborah C. Silverstein

FLUID THERAPY
*in **dogs** and **cats***

second edition

Fluid Therapy in dogs and cats - Second Edition
Fabio Viganò, Deborah C. Silverstein
©2023 Edra Publishing – All rights reserved

ISBN: 978-1-957260-25-9
eISBN: 978-1-957260-32-7

Book Publishing Manager: Costanza Smeraldi, Edra S.p.A.
Project Manager: Elisa Bechi
Paper, Printing and Binding Manager: Paolo Ficicchia, Edra S.p.A.
Cover: Ursula Giusti, Edra S.p.A.
Copyediting and Layout: Grupo Asis, Zaragoza, Spain

The rights of translation, electronic storage, reproduction or total or partial adaptation by any means (including microfilms and photostatic copies), are reserved for all countries. No part of this publication may be reproduced, stored in a retrieval system, or transmitted in any form or by any means, electronic, mechanical, photocopying, recording or otherwise, without permission in writing from the Publisher.
Knowledge and best practice in this field are constantly changing: As new research and experience broaden our knowledge, changes in practice, treatment, and drug therapy may become necessary or appropriate. Readers are advised to check the most current information provided (i) or procedures featured or (ii) by the manufacturer of each product to be administered to verify the recommended dose or formula, the method and duration of administration, and contraindications.
It is the responsibility of the practitioners, relying on their own experience and knowledge of the patient, to make diagnoses, to determine dosages and the best treatment for each individual patient, and to take all appropriate safety precautions. To the fullest extent of the law, neither the Publisher nor the Editors assume any liability for any injury and/ or damage to persons or property arising out of or related to any use of the material contained in this book.
This publication contains the author's opinions and is intended to provide precise and accurate information. The processing of the texts, even if taken care of with scrupulous attention, cannot entail specific responsibilities for the author and / or the publisher for any errors or inaccuracies. Readers should be aware that websites listed in this work may have changed or disappeared between when this work was written and when it is read. The Publisher has made every effort to obtain and cite the exact sources of the illustrations. If in some cases he has not been able to find the right holders, he is available to remedy any inadvertent omissions or errors in the references cited. Product or corporate names may be trademarks or registered trademarks, and are used only for identification and explanation without intent to infringe. All registered trademarks mentioned belong to their legitimate owners.

Edra Publishing US LLC
3309 Northlake Boulevard, Suite 203
Palm Beach Gardens, FL, 33403
EIN: 844113980
info@edrapublishing.com
www.edrapublishing.com

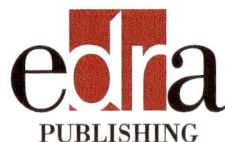

Printed in Italy by LegoDigit Srl., Lavis (TN) - February 2023

Authors

Fabio Viganò, DVM, Cert. Emergency Medicine and Surgery, Specialist in Small Animal Diseases, ECVECC AM
Clinica Veterinaria San Giorgio, San Giorgio su Legnano (Italy)

Deborah C. Silverstein, DVM, DACVECC
Department of Clinical Sciences and Advanced Medicine
University of Pennsylvania School of Veterinary Medicine
Philadelphia, Pennsylvania (USA)

Contributors

Brett Montague, DVM
Department of Clinical Sciences and Advanced Medicine
University of Pennsylvania School of Veterinary Medicine
Philadelphia, Pennsylvania (USA)

Corinna Uboldi, DVM
Clinica Veterinaria San Giorgio, San Giorgio su Legnano (Italy)

Introduction

Fluid therapy is one of the most widely used and necessary therapies for critically ill patients and those who are not able to hydrate and feed themselves spontaneously. This handbook, enriched by the contribution of two specialists, Deborah Silverstein and Brett Montague, to whom I am sincerely grateful, summarizes the fundamentals for understanding the water and electrolyte requirements of critical patients, the types of fluids that can be administered, and the consequences that a decision may entail.

From a scientific point of view, this volume is published at a particularly relevant time, with the recent developments in orthogonal polarization spectral imaging; the advancements in hemodynamics, which have made it possible to assess the real efficacy of therapy and the side effects fluids can produce if not provided correctly; and the evidence-based advances that have changed the way fluid therapy in both human and veterinary medicine is now provided, which is very different from how it had been performed over the past 30 years.

Far from being an exact science, fluid therapy is based on constant observation and continuous analysis in order to understand how it should be provided, monitor its effects, assess its efficacy, and anticipate possible collateral effects due to inappropriate administration.

Indeed, the history of fluid therapy provides many examples of events that have resulted in serious injuries and even the death of critical and noncritical patients; therefore, it has always been the subject of discussion and reevaluation based on recent discoveries, with regulatory changes implemented by international health authorities.

An attempt has been made in this book to address the topics homogeneously, following a functional approach for readers.

Chapter 1 sets out the fundamental concepts of fluid therapy, such as the principles of hemodynamics and the compartmentalization of fluids in the body. Understanding the "movement" of water in the body makes it possible to predict where the administered fluids will be distributed, in which compartments the water and electrolyte balance will be restored, and, consequently, what type of fluids should be administered. The fundamentals of hemodynamics discussed in the chapter provide information on the methods that can be used to assess the status of the cardiocirculatory activity and monitor the effects of the fluid therapy provided to a specific patient at a given moment, dose and frequency, and with a certain mode of administration.

Chapter 2 discusses the acid–base balance and explains, in a clear way, the principles of chemistry of organic and inorganic fluids, so that even veterinarians new to this discipline can assess possible acid–base alterations and choose the most appropriate treatments for each patient.

Introduction

Chapter 3 shows all the different types of fluids available and when to administer them to maintain the hydration status and provide fluid resuscitation. Even today, an agreement on the volumes and types of fluids to be administered in these two situations has not yet been reached by the scientific community.

Chapter 4 examines the electrolyte disorders that very frequently follow water imbalances: knowing which electrolytes are most commonly involved, the consequences that an alteration in their concentration may have, and how such imbalances can be corrected are the main objectives of fluid therapy.

Chapter 5 addresses hemorrhagic shock and discusses the management of critically ill patients in order to speed up triage times and find the most appropriate therapy. This chapter sets out, in a very clear manner, the basic information needed to recognize what the patient is suffering from, the consequences, and possible treatment strategies.

Finally, Chapter 6 deals with the correlation between microcirculation and fluid therapy: understanding the microcirculatory hemodynamic alterations that may occur and being able to recognize them are two fundamental steps in choosing the appropriate fluid therapy.

Every chapter ends with a clinical case, which is useful for putting into practice what has been explained in the text.

This book is aimed at all the veterinarians who are new to fluid therapy, as well as at experienced practitioners who are used to dealing with emergency patients and who, after the latest findings in this field, are interested in expanding their knowledge.

Fabio Viganò

Table of contents

1. Fundamentals of Fluid Therapy, Hemodynamics and Compartmentalization of Fluids in the Body 1
Fabio Viganò

Introduction	3
Dynamics and hemodynamics of fluid compartments	4
Water	4
Blood volume and cardiac output	5
Parameters to evaluate the hemodynamic response	8
Blood volume	13
Evaluation of cardiac output and stroke volume	13
Central venous pressure and pulmonary artery occlusion pressure	14
Clinical hemodynamic monitoring	15
Water distribution in the body	16
Osmotic pressure	16
Colloid oncotic pressure	18
Glycocalyx	19
Clinical consequences of the glycocalyx model	22
■ Clinical Case. Dehydrated dog with respiratory alkalosis	27

2. Acid–Base Disorders 31
Fabio Viganò

Introduction	33
Chemical species involved in the acid–base balance	33
Traditional approach	35
Blood gas analyzers	36
Interpretation of blood gas analysis	38
Primary disorder	38
Compensatory responses	38
Base excess (BE)	41
Anion gap (AG)	41
Total oxygen content (CaO_2)	43
Oxygen parameters to evaluate the effectiveness of oxygenation	44
Rule of 5	47
Rule of 120	47
Strong ion theory (Stewart's approach)	47
Chemical species involved	47

Table of contents

Dependent and independent variables 51
Examples of pH variations according to the nontraditional approach 51
Fluid therapy and SID 52
Clinical case, example 53
Strong ion gap (SIG) 55
Correction of acid–base disorders 55
   Metabolic acidosis 56
   Metabolic alkalosis 57
   Respiratory acidosis 59
   Respiratory alkalosis 61
   Mixed disorders 61

■ Clinical Case.
   The cat who couldn't urinate 63

3. Fluids: when and how to administer them 69
Fabio Viganò

Introduction 71
Daily intravenous fluid therapy 71
   Daily water requirements 72
   Hypotonic solutions 73
   Antidiuretic hormone and fluid therapy 76
Fluid therapy under general anesthesia 77
Daily fluid therapy 77
   Hydration 78
   Calculation of daily fluid therapy 79
Hemodynamic monitoring 80
   Heart rate and cardiac output 81
   Pulse quality 82
   Capillary refill time (CRT) 83
   Mucous membrane color 84
   Body temperature 84
   Jugular vein distension 85
   Urine production 86
   Parameters to evaluate the hemodynamic status 86
   Invasive blood pressure (IBP) measurement 92
   Measurement of lactatemia 96
Fluid resuscitation 97
   Goal-directed therapy 98
   ROSE model (Resuscitation, Optimization, Stabilization, Evacuation) 104
Crystalloids 106

Isotonic solutions	110
Hypertonic solutions	111
Colloids	112
Synthetic colloids	113
Natural colloids	115

■ Clinical Case.
　Consequences of gastroenteritis 121

4. Electrolyte Disorders 127
Fabio Viganò, Corinna Uboldi

Introduction	129
Osmosis	130
Osmolarity and osmolality	131
Sodium	132
Hyponatremia	135
Hypernatremia	139
Potassium	142
Hypokalemia	143
Hyperkalemia	144
Calcium	147
Hypocalcemia	149
Hypercalcemia	151
Phosphorus	153
Hyperphosphatemia	153
Hypophosphatemia	154
Chloride	156
Hyperchloremia	156
Hypochloremia	157
Magnesium	158
Hypomagnesemia	159
Hypermagnesemia	161

■ Clinical Case.
　Electrolyte and acid–base imbalances during vomiting 163

5. Hemorrhagic Shock 169
Brett Montague, Deborah C. Silverstein

Introduction	171
Pathophysiology of hemorrhagic shock	171
Compensatory shock	172

Table of contents

Early decompensatory shock 173
Late decompensatory shock 173
Metabolic sequelae of hemorrhagic shock 175
Etiology of hemorrhagic shock 176
Diagnosis 177
    Laboratory data 177
    Monitoring 177
    Shock index 178
    Ultrasonography 178
Clinical management 179
    Triage 179
    Hypotensive resuscitation 179
    Fluid therapy in hemorrhagic shock 180
Postresuscitation care 188
    Reperfusion injury 188
    Trauma-induced coagulopathy 188

■ Clinical Case.
    Hemorrhagic shock following a ruptured hepatocellular carcinoma 191

6. The Microcirculation and Fluid Therapy 195
Deborah C. Silverstein

Introduction 197
Structure and function of the microcirculation 197
Microvascular perfusion – systemic control 198
Microvascular perfusion – local control 201
Microvascular changes with trauma and hemorrhagic shock 202
Microvascular changes with sepsis 203
Monitoring of the microcirculation vs. macrocirculation 204
Effects of fluid resuscitation on the microcirculation in trauma
and hemorrhagic shock 207
Effects of fluid resuscitation on the microcirculation in sepsis 208
Conclusion 209

■ Clinical Case.
    Microcirculatory changes in a dog with sepsis secondary to bite wounds 217

Subject Index 221

Fundamentals of Fluid Therapy, Hemodynamics and Compartmentalization of Fluids in the Body

CHAPTER 1

Fabio Viganò

Introduction

Fluid therapy has traditionally been used for various purposes and administered by medical staff based on empirical knowledge and mathematical formulas, without a full understanding or appreciation that fluids can be considered drugs. The success or failure of the entire patient's treatment plan can depend on the adequate or ill-suited use of fluids, for example, in terms of duration of administration, type and delivery method. The aim of evidence-based medicine (EBM) should be to resolve such issues and point to the most effective procedure. EBM in human medicine does not provide clear guidance since results have been unclear and at times conflicting. In veterinary medicine, the relatively low number of patients and the absence of large-scale studies have not allowed EBM data to be collected and analyzed. Fluid therapy in veterinary medicine was therefore developed on guidelines based on human medicine. This type of approach can be the cause of errors that prove difficult to identify since our patients' hemodynamics are rarely accurately monitored and their water and electrolyte balance is not recorded.

Another factor that hampers data collection in veterinary medicine is the difficulty in defining clear guidelines. Many veterinary clinics may not be able to follow them due to a lack of financial resources (clinic or patient's owner) or technological resources (necessary equipment). Moreover, the conditions of many critical patients cannot be fully studied as all treatments or analyses must be stopped once the owner asks for their animals to be euthanized. These are the main reasons why there are so few veterinary clinics capable of collecting EBM data that can be used to improve fluid therapy and better understand the patients' conditions (Box 1.1). The scarcity of such data in small animals and the discrepancy between the information, conclusions, and guidelines can be the cause of basic mistakes, and the fluid therapy provided may therefore not be in line with the patients' needs. To reduce such mistakes and to correctly evaluate the inefficacy and the strengths and weaknesses of fluid therapy, it is necessary to carefully monitor the patient's hemodynamics as well as osmotically and oncotically active molecules.

Chapter 1 ◆ Fundamentals of Fluid Therapy and Hemodynamics

Box 1.1	Fluid therapy indications

- Maintenance of hydration
- Restoration of lost fluids
- Restoration of blood flow
- Drug administration
- Hemodynamic support

Dynamics and hemodynamics of fluid compartments

The infusion of water-based solutions in the body can restore, expand or contract one or more body fluid compartments. Knowing the structure of the vascular wall and understanding how different types of fluids behave in different compartments are the first and most fundamental steps to be able to decide on which fluids should be administered and in what amounts.

Water

Some isotopes—both radioactive and nonradioactive, such as tritium and deuterium—can be used to quantify the amount of water present in an organism. It can take an expert operator up to 3 hours to complete the procedure, which makes it impractical from a clinical point of view. The process used to quantify the plasma volume is just as complex and difficult. It entails the administration of iodinated albumin followed by the collection of 3–4 blood samples (every 10 minutes for 40 minutes). This methodology is not considered accurate, and the value is estimated at 0.91 that of humans [1].

To calculate the red blood cell mass, tracers such as chromium or technetium can be used. Carbon monoxide, which is not a tracer but is toxic, can also be used. The volume of water in the interstitial and intracellular spaces cannot be measured using tracing molecules and is therefore calculated by subtracting the plasma volume and the ECF (extracellular fluid) from the total water measured.

These methods may be more accurate than static and dynamic clinical evaluations but are more complex and difficult to perform in clinical practice. For this reason, they tend to be preferred for research and are not part of the standard practices of most veterinary clinics. In addition, to correctly perform these procedures, the patient's hemodynamics must be stable, which is difficult to achieve when patients are in critical condition. The redistribution of crystalloid fluids takes about 30 minutes, which makes precise measurements very impractical.

For the above reasons, it is common practice to use a clinical estimation of the amount of water in the body (hydration levels, see Chapter 3), which is imprecise and subjective.

Blood volume and cardiac output

Blood volume (BV) and cardiac output (CO) can be measured with methods that can be used in clinics and with critical patients. One such method is PiCCO (pulse contour cardiac output), which requires correct catheterization of a major artery (e.g., the femoral artery) and the placement of a central venous line. The arterial catheter is inserted using the Seldinger technique and is equipped with a thermistor and a light, which allows continuous arterial pressure measurement. A standard central venous catheter is used, but it is connected to a sensor that measures temperature. The pulse contour in its systolic phase provides an estimation of the stroke volume (SV), which, when multiplied by the heart rate, gives the CO. SV is a very useful parameter to monitor increases in CO following fluid therapy to restore the circulating volume in patients that are "fluid responders". Fluid responders are defined as such when a single bolus of fluids is enough to improve the CO or any other parameter used to determine whether a patient is in the ascending part of the Frank–Sterling curve (see Chapter 3, Figure 3.8). The technique requires calibration to measure the patient's vascular *compliance*.

Thanks to thermodilution, the instrument can measure the difference between the temperature of the fluid when injected (typically, saline or 5% glucose solution at 0–4 °C) and that when it comes out of the catheter. This technique provides information on cardiac performance, global end-diastolic volume (GEDV), intrathoracic total blood volume (ITBV), extra vascular lung water (EVLW), and cardiac functionality index (CFI). The instrument can also calculate stroke volume variation (SVV) and systemic vascular resistance (SVR). This technique is difficult to perform in small-sized animals and in those with arrhythmias or aortic insufficiency, but it does not require a pulmonary arterial catheter, is quick to complete, and provides sufficient information on the pulse.

Another method to obtain information on blood volume (BV) is lithium dilution cardiac output (LiDCO), which includes two procedures: the analysis of the pressure curve (Pulse CO System) and lithium thermodilution (LiDCO System). The Pulse CO algorithm is based on the correlation between the strength of the pulse and the net output and turns the pressure/time curve into a volume/time curve. This method only measures variations in the SV, not its magnitude. The LiDCO system uses lithium thermodilution. The ion is administered in a bolus in either a peripheral or central

Chapter 1 ◆ Fundamentals of Fluid Therapy and Hemodynamics

vein; a sensor is then inserted into a peripheral arterial line to measure its dilution and thus the CO. This method can use both peripheral venous and peripheral arterial blood vessels. LiDCO, as opposed to PiCCO, can measure pulse pressure variation (PPV). Both methods ensure the correct measurement of the patient's CO and response to fluid administration, and of the hemodynamic variations caused by the positive-pressure ventilation.

LiDCO measures the invasive blood pressure (IBP), SV, CO, PPV, SVV and SVR and has the advantage of being minimally invasive (peripheral vascular lines) and provides continuous information on hemodynamics. The major disadvantages of this technique are that the blood that comes into contact with the lithium electrode is toxic, lithium interferes with some drugs (e.g., muscle relaxants), instruments have to be correctly calibrated from the beginning, results may be unreliable in patients with intracardiac shunts, and the values can be altered by severe aortic regurgitation and aortic counterpulsation.

Since both LiDCO and PiCCO are difficult procedures to perform, other techniques have been developed to monitor the dynamic parameters that depend on the blood volume and effectiveness of fluid therapy to correct possible deficits (Box 1.2).

Another method that can be used to evaluate a patient's blood volume is the measurement of the LA/Ao (left atrium/aorta) ratio with an ultrasound scanner. This is done by obtaining a parasternal view of the heart both longitudinally and transversely. The standard values for both cats and dogs in the transverse view are 1–1.5 (Figure 1.1). In cats, a ratio between the aorta and left atrium greater than 2.5 is considered indicative an atrial pathology.

In patients with clinical signs of hypovolemia, a decrease in the size of the left atrium can confirm the disease. On the other hand, an increase in the left atrial diameter with no retrograde congestive heart failure or cardiomyopathy confirms hypervolemia.

An examination of the cardiac chambers in the long- and short-axis views can be useful to diagnose hyper- or hypovolemia. A skilled operator capable of performing ultrasound scans in emergency medicine can easily notice an increase in the size of the cardiac chambers and therefore roughly evaluate the total blood flow (Figures 1.2 and 1.3).

Box 1.2 — **Methods to assess cardiac output with calibration**

- PiCCO (pulse contour cardiac output)
- LiDCO (lithium dilution cardiac output)

Chapter 1 ◆ Fundamentals of Fluid Therapy and Hemodynamics

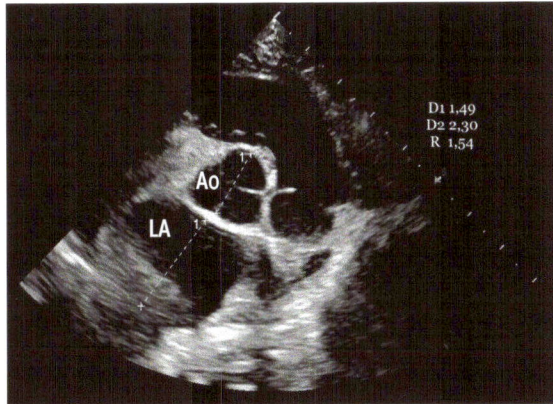

Figure 1.1 LA/Ao ratio. Parasternal transverse transaortic view of the heart (aortic ratio: LA size divided by Ao diameter). LA, left atrium; Ao, aorta.

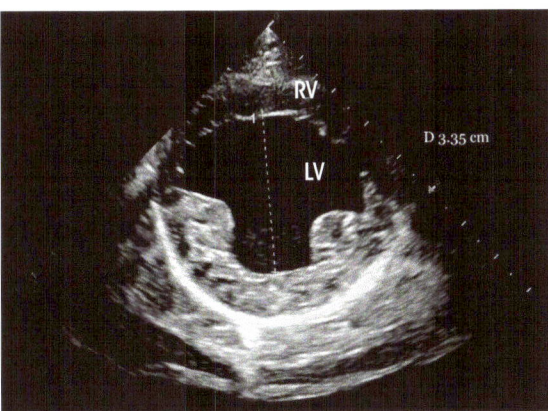

Figure 1.2 Short-axis view. In the short-axis view, it is possible to measure the left ventricular internal size when the papillary muscles are visualized at the end of diastole. RV, right ventricle; LV, left ventricle.

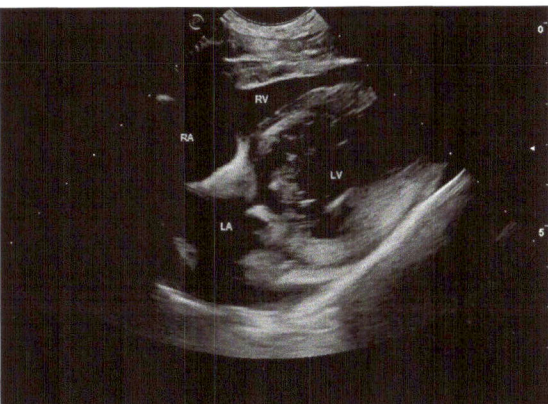

Figure 1.3 Long-axis four-chamber view. The long-axis view is useful to evaluate the size of cardiac chambers. RV, right ventricle; LV, left ventricle; RA, right atrium; LA, left atrium.

Chapter 1 ◆ Fundamentals of Fluid Therapy and Hemodynamics

Parameters to evaluate the hemodynamic response

The parameters used to measure "fluid responsiveness" are divided into dynamic and static parameters (Box 1.3). Dynamic parameters are useful to assess whether a patient is in the ascending part of the Frank–Sterling curve (see Chapter 3, Figure 3.8) and is therefore responsive to fluid therapy, or whether it is in the flat part of the curve, which could suggest no response to emergency fluid therapy and a possible circulatory overload. Static parameters, if measured at regular intervals, can provide a trend of the hemodynamic response.

Two typical examples of dynamic parameters are CO and SV measured at regular intervals over time. Unfortunately, the measurement of both parameters, in veterinary medicine, is only performed in research centers and cannot be part of the clinical routine because of the invasive nature of the procedure, the fact that only specialized clinicians can perform it, and the cost of the whole process. In veterinary medicine, it is possible to use methods that can repeatedly and accurately measure parameters correlated with CO and SV; these must precisely measure variations caused by emergency fluid therapy but should not be skewed by factors other than the increase in preload. Point-of-care ultrasound (POCUS) scans can measure the LA/Ao ratio, the diameter of the caudal vena cava (CVC), and the collapsibility index of the caudal vena cava (CVC_{CI}).

The patient's heart rate (HR) can also be useful to identify fluid responders. Unfortunately, the HR can be influenced by factors such as pain, endogenous or exogenous catecholamines, or hyperexcitement. The techniques that use POCUS can be quickly learned, depending on the operators' familiarity with the instrument.

The CVC diameter can be measured in three specific views: suprailiac, right intercostal, and subxiphoid. The latter view is where the measurement is most dependent

Box 1.3	Hemodynamic parameters: static and dynamic
Static	**Dynamic**
Clinical history	
Clinical examination	Clinical evaluation, dynamic if repeated
Thoracic X-ray	SVV
CVP	PPV
PCWP	Esophageal Doppler
Bioimpedance	CVC
	End expiratory occlusion

Chapter 1 ◆ Fundamentals of Fluid Therapy and Hemodynamics

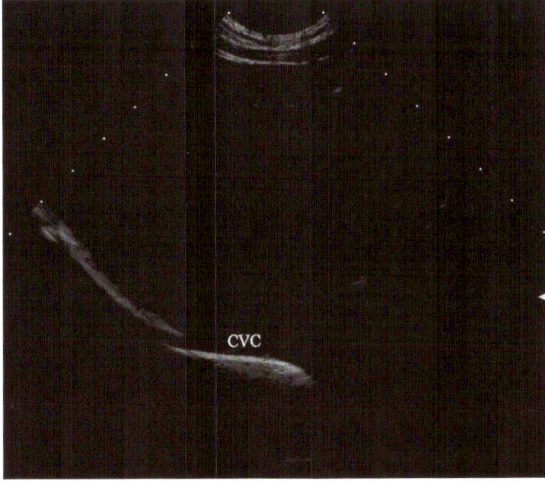

Figure 1.4. The subxiphoid view shows a normal CVC as it crosses the diaphragm. CVC, caudal vena cava.

on the operator's skill. The subxiphoid view is the easiest to obtain: the probe must be positioned longitudinally, below the xiphoid cartilage and pointing towards the cranium, so as to show the diaphragm. The probe is then oriented to show the CVC as it crosses the diaphragm (Figure 1.4). This method is very quick and easy and can be performed during the abdominal FAST (AFAST) without affecting the procedure.

The right intercostal (also called hepatic) view is obtained by positioning the probe parallel to the ribs, more precisely at the 10th–12th intercostal space, and then by moving the probe from the hypaxial muscles towards the ventral part of the thorax. If only the lung is visible, the probe should be moved down one or more intercostal spaces. If only the right kidney is visible, the probe should be moved up. The optimal position allows the CVC, the portal vein, and the aorta to be seen at the same time (Figure 1.5) just below the hypaxial muscles, close to the proximal part of the rib. When air is present, the probe should be moved down in order to correctly see the CVC. It is necessary that both the CVC and the aorta are visible at the same time.

The suprailiac (also called paralumbar) view is achieved by positioning the probe below the last right rib, guiding it towards the right kidney, and then performing a medial rotation until the aorta and CVC are visible (Figure 1.6). Once this is done, the probe should then be rotated to achieve a longitudinal view of the vessels, which should be parallel to each other (Figure 1.6). Variations in the CVC diameter are dictated by intra-aortic pressure variations in the two phases of respiration. During the inhalation phase, the negative pressure inside the thorax drives the blood from the abdomen towards the right atrium, causing maximum CVC diameter reduction. During the expiration phase, the opposite occurs, causing maximum CVC relaxation.

Chapter 1 ◆ Fundamentals of Fluid Therapy and Hemodynamics

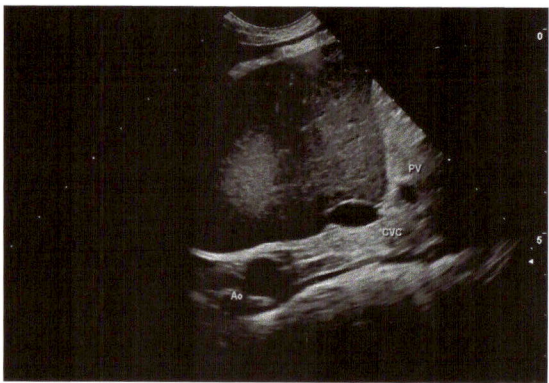

Figure 1.5 Hepatic view (right 10th–12th intercostal space) showing the CVC, aorta and portal vein. CVC, caudal vena cava; Ao, aorta; PV, portal vein.

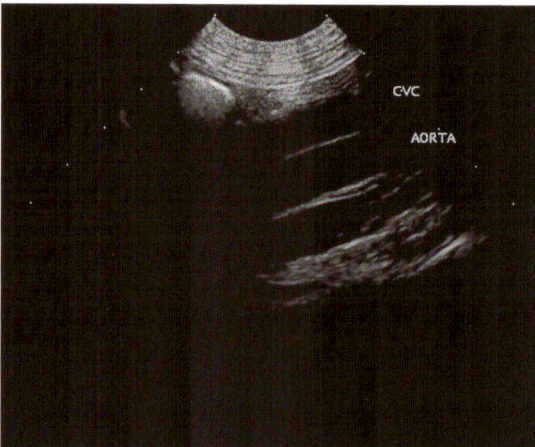

Figure 1.6. Paralumbar view (suprailiac) view of the CVC and aorta. CVC, caudal vena cava; Ao, aorta.

Hypovolemia causes the diameter of the CVC to be decreased; an increase in the CVC diameter following fluid administration demonstrates a positive response to emergency fluid therapy. This may also occur in cases of mitral valve regurgitation. The sole monitoring of the CVC diameter is not enough to measure the response to fluid therapy continuously and precisely. The variation in the CV diameter between inhalation and expiration is called CVC_{CI} and can be calculated using the following formula:

$$CVC_{CI} = (CVC_d \max - CVC_d \min)/CVC_d \max \qquad (Equation\ 1)$$

CVC_{CI}, collapsibility index of the caudal vena cava; CVC_d max, maximum diameter of the caudal vena cava; CVC_d min, minimum diameter of the caudal vena cava.

Chapter 1 ◆ Fundamentals of Fluid Therapy and Hemodynamics

Values above 50% could indicate hypervolemia, hence the risk of an increase of extravascular lung water (EVLW), congestive heart failure, or cardiac tamponade. Values below 50% are usually recorded in hypovolemic patients. The variation in the diameter of the CVC in hypovolemic patients is very low and the CVC may appear as a collapsed vein that does not expand during the respiratory cycle. In hypervolemic patients, the CVC diameter does not change and will appear as a dilated blood vessel that has lost its elasticity. A patient's response to fluid therapy can be proved if, following the administration of one or more boluses, there is relaxation of the CVC. CVC diameter measurement can be invalidated by cardiac performance, the intraabdominal and intrathoracic pressures, anxiety, tachycardia, pregnancy, physical activity, stress, obesity, diabetes, and kidney failure. This promising diagnostic tool remains to be validated through publications involving a significant number of dogs and especially cats.

A dedicated study [2] has successfully demonstrated the possibility of evaluating whether patients are fluid responders by administering a small 4 mL bolus of Ringer's lactate in 1 minute and measuring the left ventricular end-diastolic internal diameter normalized to body weight (LVIDDn), the left ventricular volume score (LVVS), the left ventricular end-diastolic volume index (EDVI), and the aortic velocity time integral (VTI). Unfortunately, this technique requires advanced skills since inaccurate measurements can lead to errors in data interpretation. The measurement of hemodynamic parameters has made the use of ultrasound in veterinary emergency medicine and intensive care increasingly important. The ultrasound scanner can be used to view the abdomen and respiratory system but also to dynamically monitor the efficacy of fluid therapy.

A new method that has to be yet validated in veterinary medicine is electrical velocimetry (EV). EV can detect CO and SVV [3] but should be studied in a sufficient number of patients, both awake and under general anesthesia. In human medicine, the dynamic parameters that can be used to identify fluid responders are SVV (stroke volume variation), SPV (systolic pressure variation) and PPV (pulse pressure variation). The correlation between BV and SPV variations is well understood [2]. PPV is also strongly correlated with SVV and is less affected by variations in SPV [3]. PPV is a more reliable parameter to measure the patient's hemodynamic response to fluid therapy than SVV, since it is measured directly and not through specific instruments that use PCA (pulse contour analysis).

Another parameter commonly used in human medicine to determine the response to fluid therapy, which is strongly correlated with PPV, is PVI (pleth variability index). PVI is an automatic, noninvasive, and continuous measurement performed by a specific instrument (Radical 7® Masimo), which can detect plethysmographic variations and hence hemodynamic variations during the respiratory cycle.

Chapter 1 ◆ Fundamentals of Fluid Therapy and Hemodynamics

Increased variations during spontaneous respiration or positive pressure ventilation (PPV) point to a reduced blood volume (i.e., preload) or increased intrathoracic pressure. PVI is a variation of PI (perfusion index) during the respiratory cycle; in human medicine, values greater than 10–15% point to a reduced blood volume and to the fact that an increased blood volume can lead to an increased CO and, therefore, to greater responsiveness to fluid therapy. PVI is inversely proportional to the blood volume, which means an increase in PVI indicates a reduction in blood flow. The higher the PVI readings, the more severe the hypovolemia.

PI is a percentage of the light intensity emitted by the diode and the light absorbed by the pulsatile arterial blood in circulation. It measures the strength of the signal and the local vasomotor tone, and its values are between 0.02% and 20%. In human medicine, values above 1% are considered normal. PI can vary depending on the patient and on where the measurement is performed. It is measured using the following formula:

$$PI = \frac{AC}{DC} \times 100 \qquad (Equation\ 2)$$

AC, infrared light absorbed by the pulsatile arterial blood; DC, light emitted by the diode and absorbed by the skin, the pulsatile arterial blood, and interposed tissues.

PVI is calculated by measuring PI over a sufficient period of time to allow one or more respiratory cycles, using the following formula:

$$PVI = \frac{PI_{max} - PI_{min}}{PI_{max}} \times 100 \qquad (Equation\ 3)$$

In human medicine, in 81% of cases, values above 14% indicate responsiveness to fluid therapy. Values below 14% indicate nonresponsiveness to fluid therapy in 100% of cases. It has also been demonstrated that the administration of fluid therapy based on the careful monitoring of PPV and PVI can improve the outcome [6] and optimize the hemodynamic condition of patients undergoing abdominal surgery [7]. The shortcomings of this monitoring method are that values may be altered in case of an increase in abdominal pressure or right-heart failure, it is necessary to have a sinus rhythm and the thorax must be closed, it has not been validated in veterinary medicine, and PI and PVI may vary in animal patients between spontaneous and controlled breathing (Box 1.4).

Chapter 1 ◆ Fundamentals of Fluid Therapy and Hemodynamics

Box 1.4	Hemodynamic response monitoring

Parameters to evaluate the hemodynamic response
- PPV (pulse pressure variation)
- PVI (pleth variability index)
- PI (perfusion index)
- Hemodynamic support

Blood volume

The measurement of BV in animal patients requires an invasive procedure that is difficult to perform. This explains why many studies are being conducted on how to evaluate BV and the response to fluid therapy through biodynamic parameters, such as the CVC diameter. The CVC has a very thin wall sensitive to internal volume variations. During the respiratory cycle, the CVC diameter varies. It should be highlighted that the venous compartment holds around 2/3 of the blood volume and that the CVC is the largest venous vessel in animals. During the inspiration phase, the negative pressure inside the thorax reduces the blood flow inside the CVC, while during the expiration phase the increase in the thoracic pressure causes a greater flow of blood into the CVC, thereby increasing its diameter. Precise measurement of the CVC during the two phases was performed in a recent study [8]. Data have highlighted that the CVC/aorta diameter ratio, measured in the lumbar region of the left kidney, can be used to evaluate BV in dogs undergoing blood transfusion. This technique could become a noninvasive method to evaluate the decrease in BV after a severe blood loss. Its significance and accuracy in cases of circulatory overload or following excessive fluid administration are not known. No similar study has been performed in cats. Some limitations of this technique are the impossibility to record data continuously, the probable unreliability when intra-abdominal pressure increases (e.g., postsurgery or when fluids are present in the abdomen cavity), and the patient's morphology.

Evaluation of cardiac output and stroke volume

A noninvasive method to measure both SV and CO is *esophageal Doppler*. This is done by inserting an ultrasound Doppler probe through the mouth into the esophagus. By measuring the diameter of the aorta and the distribution and velocity of the blood flow, the probe can evaluate the cardiac preload [9]. The main drawbacks of this technique are the need to perform general anesthesia and intubate the patient to protect the airways from gastric contents in the event of vomiting, the need to recali-

Chapter 1 ◆ Fundamentals of Fluid Therapy and Hemodynamics

brate the measurements every time, and the impossibility to monitor the parameters continuously. *Transesophageal echocardiography* is similar to esophageal doppler in terms of the parameters being measured, advantages and disadvantages, but its reliability in animals has not been validated.

Bioimpedance, a technique used in human medicine to evaluate body fluids, uses weak electrical currents that travel through tissues and are hindered by the presence of water. In human medicine, this technique has been used to evaluate both the intracellular fluid (ICF) and extracellular fluid (ECF). In veterinary medicine there are no publications on this technique in small animals. It is a static measurement of BV and, in humans, it is strongly correlated with total water, which makes it useful in treating congestive heart failure, during dialysis and terminal stage kidney failure. It is not useful to determine the intravascular volume and the response to fluid therapy [10] (Box 1.5).

Central venous pressure and pulmonary artery occlusion pressure

Central venous pressure (CVP) and *pulmonary artery occlusion pressure* (PAOP, or *pulmonary capillary wedge pressure*, PCWP) are static parameters of preload and have been used evaluate the patient's response to fluid therapy, but recent studies in veterinary and human medicine have questioned their reliability [11–13].

Their use is therefore not recommended to measure BV or as a tool to assess the response to fluid therapy in critical patients or when excessive amounts of fluids have been administered, since CVP increases over normal values only when vessel *compliance* (elasticity of venous walls, especially in large vessels) has been exceeded.

Box 1.5 — **Parameters to evaluate blood volume, cardiac output and stroke volume**

Assessment of blood volume
- POCUS (point-of-care ultrasound)
- CVC (caudal vena cava) diameter and CVC_{CI} (CVC diameter variations)

Cardiac output and stroke volume
- Esophageal Doppler
- Transesophageal echocardiography
- Bioimpedance
- Electrical velocimetry

Chapter 1 ◆ Fundamentals of Fluid Therapy and Hemodynamics

CVP is the pressure in the venous part of circulation, while mean arterial pressure (MAP) is the pressure in the arterial part of circulation. CVP is useful to detect decreases in CO in cardiogenic shock caused by insufficient preload; in these cases, a reduction in CVP indicates the need to administer fluids, while high values suggest tension pneumothorax or lung thromboembolism. CVP is also useful to manage chronic heart failure since high values cause a deterioration of kidney functions. CVP could be considered as the interstitial compartment's "exit" pressure.

Clinical hemodynamic monitoring

When it is not possible to assess hemodynamic parameters and the efficacy of fluid therapy or vasoactive amines through dynamic monitoring with POCUS or an invasive method, it is advisable to request the patient's history and to repeatedly perform *clinical* (Chapter 3) and lab *monitoring* in order to determine at the very least the following parameters:
- state of consciousness;
- capillary refill time and mucous membrane color;
- heart rate;
- body temperature;
- jugular vein relaxation;
- mean arterial pressure and systolic arterial pressure;
- pulse (characteristics and quality);
- skin (elasticity, turgor, dryness, temperature at extremities);
- shock index (HR/SAP, ≥0.9 unfavorable prognosis);
- peripheral edema;
- urine production and its specific weight;
- lactatemia;
- urea or creatinine.

Some of these parameters (pulse, state of consciousness, skin, CRT) are subjective and not absolute points of reference. The values of such parameters should be explained when choosing the therapy, in the medical report, and at shift changes to reduce the possibility of mistakes and so clinicians and the paramedical staff can make decisions based on the same standards. Unfortunately, clinical monitoring is not reliable to evaluate BV and it cannot identify fluid responders, even if an improvement in these parameters would indicate a positive response to the treatment. The more clinical parameters are recorded, the more accurate they will be in monitoring the hemodynamic status.

Chapter 1 ◆ Fundamentals of Fluid Therapy and Hemodynamics

Water distribution in the body

Water makes up around 60% of the total body weight. ECF is the water present in the intravascular and interstitial compartments, while ICF (Figure 1.1) is intracellular water.

The fluid compartments and the water contained in them are:
- intracellular (67%, about 0.4 L/kg);
- interstitial (25%, about 0.13 L/kg);
- intravascular (8%, about 0.06 L/kg).

Fluid therapy should not solely be based on the quantity of water present in the body in normal conditions and on the water lost by the organism. It should also take into consideration the patient's hemodynamic parameters and their water and electrolyte balance just before fluid administration. As a matter of fact, any conditions prior to the body losing fluids and alterations caused by the pathological process can change the patient's needs, and the composition and amount of fluids necessary and how they should be administered. Two patients suffering from the same pathology causing dehydration or compromising the efficacy of blood circulation may have different needs. For example, a patient suffering from chronic congestive heart failure caused by mitral regurgitation will have a limited tolerance to a rapid infusion of large volumes of crystalloids compared to a patient whose hemodynamic parameters are not affected by increases in pulmonary arterial pressure. Water moves in the three compartments according to osmotic and oncotic gradients. The walls dividing the three compartments are the vascular and cellular walls (see Figure 1.7). The first is permeable to water and small solutes such as sodium, chloride and potassium (the diameter of sodium is 2–3 angstroms [Å], chlorine 2 Å and potassium about 2.2 Å). The smaller pores of the vascular membrane have a diameter of about 40–45 Å. The cellular wall, on the other hand, is only permeable to water (Box 1.6).

Osmotic pressure

Osmotic pressure is exerted by small particles such as sodium, urea, and glucose, while oncotic pressure is exerted by large molecules, such as proteins and hydroxyethyl starches.

The osmotic pressure can be calculated using the formula below (Box 1.7):

$$\text{Osm} = 2 \times [\text{Na}^+] + \text{glucose (mg/dL)}/18 + \text{BUN (mg/dL)}/2.8 \qquad \textit{(Equation 3)}$$

Normal osmotic values are about 310 mOsm/L in dogs and 320 mOsm/L in cats. These can be measured with a specific tool, the osmometer. The formula also shows

Chapter 1 ◆ Fundamentals of Fluid Therapy and Hemodynamics

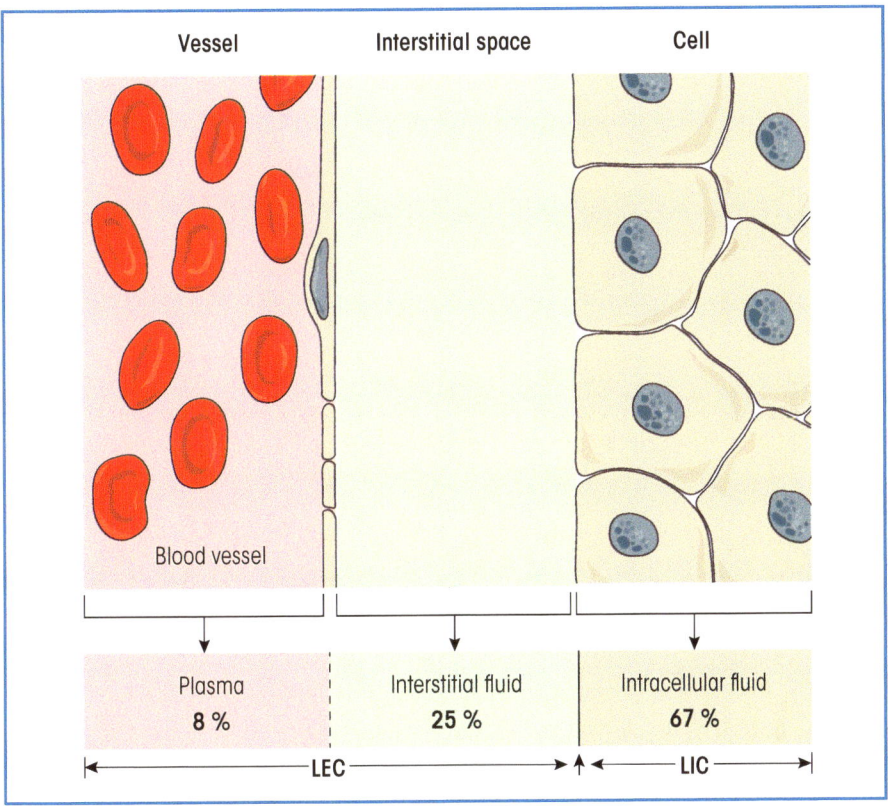

Figure 1.7 Fluid compartments. ECF, extracellular fluid; ICF, intracellular fluid.

Box 1.6	Distribution of water in the organism

Water makes up around 60% of the total body weight, divided in:
- intracellular: 67%, about 0.4 L/kg
- interstitial: 25%, about 0.13 L/kg
- intravascular: 8%, about 0.06 L/kg

that osmotic pressure is mostly exerted by chloride (about 140 times 2) and, to a lesser extent, by glucose (about 100 divided by 18) and nonprotein nitrogen (about 25 divided by 2.8).

Chapter 1 ◆ Fundamentals of Fluid Therapy and Hemodynamics

> **Box 1.7** — **Osmotic and oncotic pressure formulas**
>
> **Osmotic pressure**
> Osm = 2 [Na⁺] + glucose (mg/dL)/18 + BUN (mg/dL)/2.8
>
> **Oncotic pressure**
> COP = (2.1 × PT) + (0.16 × PT) + (0.09 × PT)
>
> BUN (blood urea nitrogen), azotemia; COP, osmotic colloid pressure; [Na⁺], concentration of sodium in the blood; Osm, blood osmolality; PT, total proteins.

Following the law of mass action, an increase in osmotic pressure in one of the compartments separated by a semipermeable membrane causes the movement of water from the compartment with a lower concentration towards the compartment with a higher concentration, in an attempt to balance the system in terms of particles present on both sides of the membrane. Particles with an electric charge must be present in equal amounts in compartments divided by a semipermeable membrane. The osmotic pressure is therefore driven by the number of active particles present in the solute inside the compartment.

For example, in cases of kidney failure with an increase in azotemia, or in cases of hyperosmolar syndrome or illnesses such as diabetes mellitus with an increase in blood glucose, the osmotic pressure inside in the intravascular (IV) compartment will increase, causing water to move towards this compartment and therefore dehydration of the extravascular compartment. For the same reason, when the sodium concentration inside the IV compartment increases (e.g., after the intravenous administration of a hypertonic saline solution), water moves from the extravascular compartment towards the IV compartment, causing an increase in blood volume.

The same osmotic gradient can be exerted by a semipermeable membrane, such as a cell wall, when the concentration of sodium or other osmotically active molecules increases inside the cell. In these cases, the amount of water increases and may cause cellular edema. When this happens inside the brain, alterations of the state of consciousness may occur, such as stupor, coma or death. Unlike cellular walls, vascular walls allow the passage of some proteins, causing a continuous exchange of proteins between the intravascular and extravascular compartments, with a continuous flow of fluids through the capillary membranes between the compartments. This flow is called transcapillary escape rate (TER), and generally refers to albumin.

Colloid oncotic pressure

The oncotic gradient is created by the large molecules inside the IV compartment. All molecules larger than 10 000 dalton can increase **colloid oncotic pressure** (COP).

Chapter 1 ◆ Fundamentals of Fluid Therapy and Hemodynamics

The molecules naturally present in the IV compartment and capable of generating this gradient are albumins, globulins, and fibrinogen. Albumin is the smallest and its molecular mass is 69 000 dalton and diameter about 140 Å, but it is also the most abundant. The oncotic gradient generated by large molecules is calculated with a formula derived from Starling's law, and published in 1896:

$$Jv = Kf (P_c - Pi_f) - \sigma (\pi_c - \pi_{if}) - Q \text{ lymph} \quad (Equation\ 4)$$

Jv, transvascular flow; Kf, filtration coefficient; P_c, capillary hydrostatic pressure; P_{if}, interstitial hydrostatic pressure; π_c, COP plasma; π_{if}, interstitial COP; σ, reflection coefficient; Q lymph, lymphatic drainage.

This formula suggested that the main driver of fluid movement (Jv) to and from the IV compartment was hydrostatic pressure (intravascular and interstitial). Hydrostatic pressure was therefore the main driver of an increase in Jv, and for the same reason decreases in COP would increase Jv. Conversely, increases in COP would lead to movement of fluids from the extravascular space towards the intravascular space. This has led to treatments that were not producing the expected results. For example, the administration of solutions containing albumin did not lead to water reabsorption from the interstitial sapce, while increases in hydrostatic pressure were responsible for a short-term increase of Jv, which did not occur in a state of hemodynamic equilibrium.

Thanks to studies on the vascular wall with the use of electronic microscopy (e.g., using the orthonormalization method in ghost imaging) and dilution techniques with dextran or indocyanine green, it was possible to observe the internal surface of the vascular endothelium, where a viscous substance called glycocalyx was found, the influence of which on Jv has been evaluated.

Glycocalyx

The **glycocalyx** is a layer of glycoproteins and proteoglycans attached to the endoluminal surface of blood vessels and negatively charged. The *core* is made up of proteoglycans (syndecan, glypican, and versican) to which long sulphate molecules (such as heparan, dermatan, hyaluronic acid, and chondroitin sulfate) attach to create a surface resembling marine algae (Figure 1.8).

Molecules positioned in this way dynamically interact with coagulation factors and with the complement system/cascade that regulates the permeability of blood vessels. The small space just below the glycocalyx is called sub-glycocalyx. It has its own oncotic pressure (π_{sg}), mostly exerted by albumin, which creates a gradient

Chapter 1 ◆ Fundamentals of Fluid Therapy and Hemodynamics

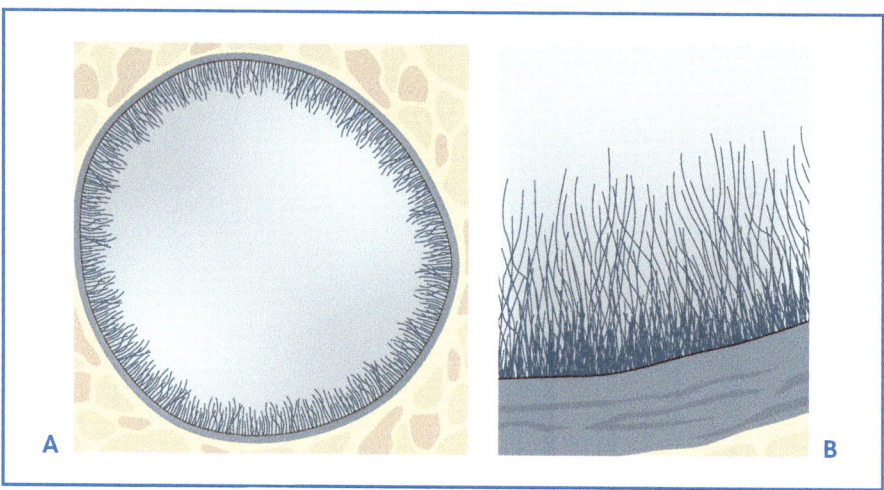

Figure 1.8 Representation of an electronic microscope scan of the glycocalyx. **(A)** Section of a vessel with intact glycocalyx. **(B)** Detail of the glycocalyx.

between the endoluminal oncotic pressure and the sub-glycocalyx. The sub-glycocalyx oncotic pressure contributes to control Jv.

The glycocalyx covers endothelial receptors as well as other molecules attached to the endothelial membranes. Its average thickness is about 2 µm and it stretches over a surface of about 350 m². In humans, it has a volume of about 1700 mL and the fluids it contains are not part of the total circulating volume. It is thicker in large vessels (8 µm) and thinner in small vessels (0.2 µm). The glycocalyx is semipermeable to albumin, to molecules with a molecular weight below 70 kDa, and to dextran; it is impermeable to red blood cells (RBCs).

The glycocalyx present in most capillaries acts like a plasma filter for large molecules and is permeable to water. The glycocalyx divides the intravascular space in three areas (Figure 1.9): the central area (plasma volume), a noncirculating fluid component and the RBCs.

The vascular wall is different in the capillaries of the various tissues, which is why crystalloids are useful in increasing blood volume: because of their structure, they do not exit the capillaries of tissues (e.g., the brain, muscles, lungs, connective tissues and capsules of parenchymatous organs) and therefore increase the intravascular space. Conversely, when excessive fluids are administered and there is damage to the vessel wall, crystalloids can distribute to the ECF, causing interstitial edema and a possible compartment syndrome [14].

In human anatomy, the blood vessels of the nervous system, muscles, connective tissues, and lungs are terminal vessels, while endocrine blood vessels and ves-

Chapter 1 ◆ Fundamentals of Fluid Therapy and Hemodynamics

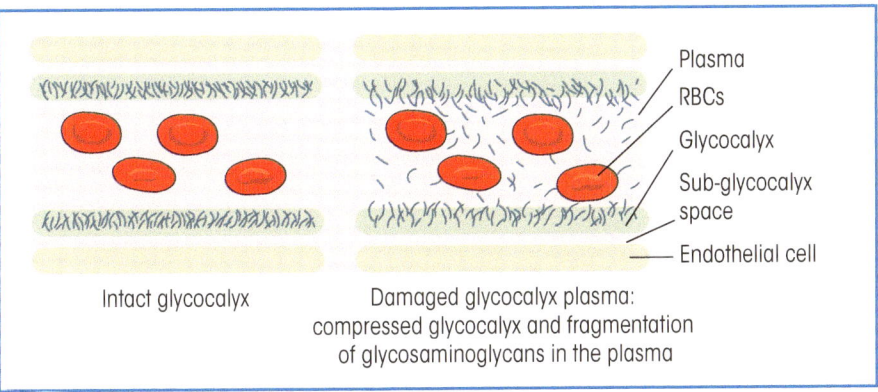

Figure 1.9 Vascular wall and glycocalyx. RBCs, red blood cells.

sels of the choroid plexus and intestinal and glomerular mucosa are fenestrated. However, the glycocalyx is not present in the blood vessels of the liver, spleen, and bone marrow, and the fenestrations they present thus allow the passage of macromolecules such as chylomicrons and lipoproteins. For this very reason, COP does not influence the flow of fluids through the vascular wall, but rather the flow depends predominantly on the hydrostatic pressure in the lymphatic system (Figure 1.10) [14].

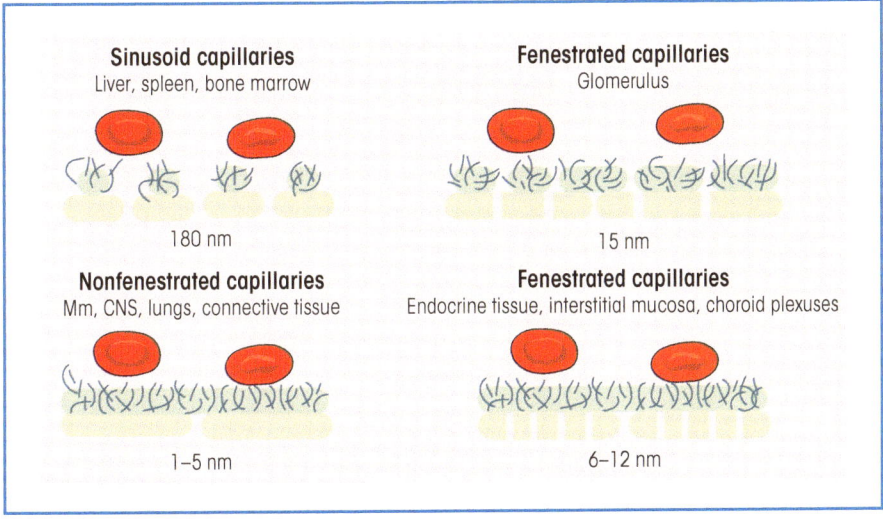

Figure 1.10 Capillary phenotypes with respective fenestration diameters.

21

According to the glycocalyx model, Jv is also influenced by the filtration coefficient (Kf), which can affect vascular permeability, since an increase in Kf helps the flow of water towards the extravascular space. Kf is the result of the total capillary surface multiplied by the hydraulic conductivity and the reflection coefficient (σ). The reflection coefficient influences the permeability of plasma proteins and when their molecular weight exceeds 70 KDa, they become impermeable, thus generating oncotic pressure. A σ equal to 1.0 indicates total impermeability of the membrane, while a σ equal to 0.0 means molecules can freely pass through the membranes. In cats and dogs, σ varies between 0.83 and 0.92. In humans, σ for albumin is approximately 0.90–0.95 in the muscles, approximately 0.50–0.65 in the lungs, and 0.8 in the intestine and subcutaneous tissue.

The Starling formula (Equation 4) was modified following the knowledge provided by the study of the vascular walls and is now known as the Michel–Weinbaum formula:

$$Jv = Kf\,[(P_c - P_i) - \sigma\,(\pi_p - \pi_{sg})] \qquad (Equation\ 5)$$

Jv, transvascular flow; Kf, filtration coefficient; P_c, capillary hydrostatic pressure; P_i, interstitial hydrostatic pressure; σ, reflection coefficient; π_p, plasma COP; π_{sg}, sub-glycocalyx COP.

Clinical consequences of the glycocalyx model

The new formula considers the COP of the sub-glycocalyx (π_{sg}) and that of the IV compartment (π_p) to be decisive, instead of the COP of the IV and interstitial spaces.

This review [15] and the study of vascular walls suggest that Jv depends predominantly on hydrostatic pressure; that an increase in COP at normal capillary pressures (20 mmHg) does not cause the reabsorption of fluids from the interstitial space; and that increases in the hydrostatic pressure (P_c) above the oncotic pressure are responsible for a linear increase in Jv, enough to drive a sudden rise in the filtration/hydrostatic pressure curve (Figure 1.11). Experimental studies conducted on the mesenteric vessels of frogs and rats have demonstrated that rapid increases in P_c cause a linear rise in Jv, but when, under conditions of hemodynamic stability, P_c was lower than π_p, there was no reabsorption of fluids from the interstitial space.

When administering fluid therapy with crystalloids, even if pulmonary capillaries have a very low P_c (between −5 mmHg and −10 mmHg), it is important, to avoid pulmonary edema, to carefully monitor the blood COP to ensure it is not excessively reduced, since this would increase the Jv and cause interstitial edema.

This new revision also demonstrates that, under normal conditions, the plasma, interstitial fluid, and lymphatic system are placed in series, and fluids continuously flow from one compartment to the other. Therefore, reabsorption occurs through the lymphatic circulation and not through the capillaries.

Chapter 1 ◆ Fundamentals of Fluid Therapy and Hemodynamics

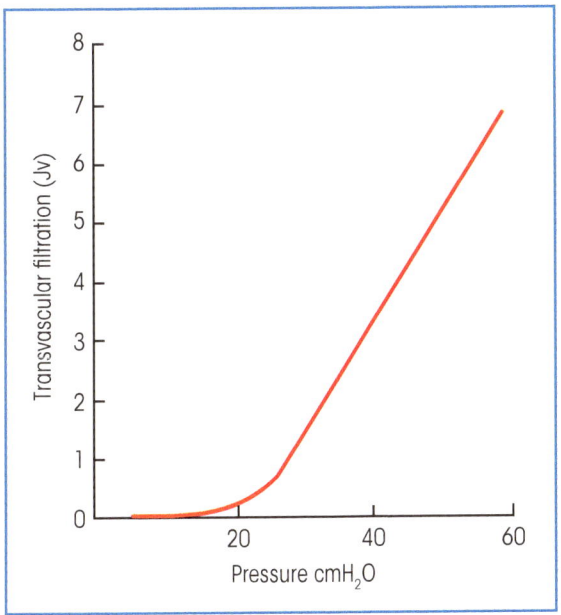

Figure 1.11 Relation between transvascular filtration (Jv) and hydrostatic pressure (P_c).

The administration of fluid therapy with colloids and crystalloids has been reconsidered in light of the new model of Jv regulation. According to Starling's hypothesis, the administration of crystalloids limits the physiological response to the simple reduction of total flow. The new interpretation shows that when endocapillary pressure (P_c) decreases (e.g., during severe blood loss), the crystalloids administered remain in the blood. This hypothesis has changed the fluids of choice (crystalloids over colloids) to be administered to patients with low blood pressure [17].

In human medicine, the glycocalyx can perform a sort of "autotransfusion" when the patient is suffering from hypotension following severe blood loss (around 750 mL). In patients with a normal blood pressure or hypertension, this phenomenon is reduced by a third to a half. The effects of this phenomenon are highest when colloid solutions are administered to patients with hypovolemia and an intact glycocalyx. The expansion of the circulating volume following the administration of colloids depends on the blood volume and the status of the glycocalyx.

When water and proteins accumulate in the interstitial space (e.g., during sepsis or as a consequence of an inflammatory disease such as systemic inflammatory response syndrome [SIRS]), excess fluids are transferred to the general circulation through the lymphatic system and only in small part through capillary reabsorption. A deficient lymphatic circulation and a rise in capillary permeability can therefore lead to an excess of proteins and fluids in the interstitial space, causing interstitial edema.

Chapter 1 ◆ Fundamentals of Fluid Therapy and Hemodynamics

Lymphatic drainage increases with a rise in muscular activity and decreases when the patient does not move. Hypovolemic patients with reduced mobility who have developed an inflammatory illness such as SIRS can more easily develop ECF edema following an increase in transvascular flow and a decrease in lymphatic drainage. Physiotherapy and muscular activity can reduce the need to administer colloid solutions since they increase drainage in the ECF space. The brain, however, lacks lymphatic drainage. In the brain, the capillary membrane is impermeable to most molecules, with the exception of water. As a matter of fact, the blood–brain barrier (BBB) is impermeable to large and small molecules (e.g., sodium and proteins).

Within the brain, the Jv predominantly depends on the hydrostatic pressure and on the blood's oncotic and osmotic pressure. For this reason, damage to the BBB, such as that caused by trauma, leads to an increase in its permeability, thus allowing the passage of small solutes, which results in an increase in Jv. This in turn leads to interstitial edema and, as a consequence, to an increase in intracranial pressure.

A loss of glycocalyx integrity (known as shedding) causes an increase in vascular permeability, especially with regard to proteins and negatively charged molecules towards the extravascular space, which leads to perivascular edema [18]. In humans, the rapid administration of crystalloids causes an increase in hyaluronic acid, which indicates damage to the glycocalyx [19,20]. Inflammatory states, sepsis, diabetes, surgery, hypertension, and trauma are often associated with damage to the glycocalyx.

Box 1.8 — Clinical consequences of the glycocalyx model

- The COP of the glycocalyx and that of the IV compartment are very important for Jv, but not the interstitial COP.
- Jv mostly depends on hydrostatic pressure.
- An increase in COP at a normal capillary pressure (20 mmHg) does not cause the absorption of fluids from the interstitial space.
- Increases in the hydrostatic pressure (P_c) greater than the oncotic pressure lead to a linear increase in Jv.
- When the total blood flow is reduced, the crystalloids administered remain in the blood flow, just like colloids.
- Water and proteins accumulated in the interstitial space are transferred to the general blood circulation through the lymphatic system.
- A loss of integrity of the glycocalyx causes and increase in vascular permeability.

COP, osmatic colloid pressure; JV, transvascular flow.

Chapter 1 ◆ Fundamentals of Fluid Therapy and Hemodynamics

Damage to the glycocalyx can be caused by inflammatory mediators such as C-reactive protein, tissue necrosis factor, the stimulation of A_3 adenosine receptors, bradykinin, and the activation of neutrophil granulocytes and mast cells. The products of the fragmentation of the glycocalyx in the blood circulation behave like proinflammatory chemotactic molecules, which contributes to the worsening of inflammatory states or inhibits counterregulation mechanisms.

Damage to the glycocalyx can be assessed in vivo with an electron microscope or by measuring the glycocalyx degradation products (e.g., syndecan 1, hyaluronic acid, heparan sulphate, and chondroitin sulphate) (Box 1.8).

References

[1] Zdolsek J, Lisander B, Hahn RG. Measuring the size of the extracellular fluid space using bromide, iohexol and sodium dilution. *Anesth Analg*. 2005;101:1770–1777.

[2] Rick JJ, Burke SS. Respiratory paradox. *South Med J*. 1978;71:1376–1378.

[3] Monnet X, Bleibtreu A, Ferre A et al. Passive leg raising and end-expiratory occlusion tests perform better than pulse pressure variation in patients with low respiratory system compliance. *Crit Care Med*. 2012;40:152–157.

[4] Natalini G, Rosano A, Taranto M et al. Arterial versus plethysmographic dynamic indices to test responsiveness for testing fluid administration in hypotensive patients: a clinical trial. *Anesth Analg*. 2006;103:1478–1484.

[5] Wenqing L, Jing D, Zifeng X et al. The pleth variability index as an indicator of the central extracellular fluid volume in mechanically ventilated patients after anesthesia induction: comparison with initial distribution volume of glucose. *Med Sci Monit*. 2014;20:386–392.

[6] Cannesson M. Arterial pressure variation and goal-directed fluid therapy. *J Cardiothorac Vasc Anesth*. 2010 Jun;24(3):487–497.

[7] Forget P, Lois F, de Kock M.Goal-directed fluid management based on the pulse oximeter-derived pleth variability index reduces lactate levels and improves fluid management. *Anesth Analg*. 2010 Oct;111(4):910–914.

[8] Cambournac M, Goy-Thollot I, Violé A, Barthélemy A. Sonographic assessment of volemia (SAV) in dogs: determination and validation of a new method. Abstract. In: *Proceedings of EVECCS*. 2017; Dublin, Ireland.

[9] Dark PM, Singer M. The validity of trans-esophageal Doppler ultrasonography as a measure of cardiac output in critically ill adults. *Intensive Care Med*. 2004;30:2060–2066.

[10] Ronco C, Kaushik M, Valle R et al. Diagnosis and management of fluid overload in heart failure and cardio-renal syndrome: the "5B Approach". *Semin Nephrol*. 2012;32:129–141.

[11] Hutchinson KM, Shaw SP. A review of central venous pressure and its reliability as a hemodynamic monitoring tool in veterinary medicine. *Top Companion Anim Med*. 2016;31(3):109–121.

Chapter 1 ◆ Fundamentals of Fluid Therapy and Hemodynamics

[12] Marik PE. Techniques for assessment of intravascular volume in critically ill patients. *J Intensive Care Med.* 2009;24(5):329–337.

[13] Kalantari K, Chang JN, Ronco C, Rosner MH. Assessment of intravascular volume status and volume responsiveness in critically ill patients. *Kidney Int.* 2013;83(6):1017–1028.

[14] Woodcock TE, Woodcock TM. Revised Starling equation and the glycocalyx model of transvascular fluid exchange: an improved paradigm for prescribing intravenous fluid therapy. *Br J Anaesth.* 2012 Mar;108(3):384–394.

[15] Levick JR, Michel CC. Microvascular fluid exchange and the revised Starling principle. *Cardiovasc Res.* 2010;27:198–210.

[16] Zhang X, Adamson RH, Curry FE, Weinbaum S. Transient regulation of transport by pericytes in venular microvessels via trapped microdomains. *Proc Natl Acad Sci USA.* 2008;105:1374–1379.

[17] Hahn RG. Volume kinetics for infusion fluids. *Anestesiology.* 2010;113;470–481.

[18] Salmon AH, Satchell SC. Endothelial glycocalyx dysfunction in diseases: albuminuria and increased microvascular permeability. *J Pathol.* 2012;226:562–574.

[19] Berg S, Engman A, Hesselvik JF, Laurent TC. Crystalloid infusion increases plasma hyaluronan. *Crit Care Med.* 1994;22:1563–1567.

[20] Berg S, Golster M, Lisander B. Albumin extravasation and tissue washout of hyaluronan after plasma volume expansion with crystalloid or hypooncotic colloid solutions. Acta *Anaesthesiol Scand.* 2002;46:166–172.

[21] Nieuwdorp M, van Haeften TW, Gouverneur MC et al. Loss of endothelial glycocalyx during acute hyperglycemia coincides with endothelial dysfunction and coagulation activation in vivo. *Diabetes.* 2006;55:480–486.

[22] Rehm M, Bruegger D, Christ F et al. Shedding of the endothelial glycocalyx in patients undergoing major vascular surgery with global and regional ischemia. *Circulation.* 2007;116:1896–1906.

[23] Nieuwdorp M, Mooij HL, Kroon J et al. Endothelial glycocalyx damage coincides with microalbuminuria in type 1 diabetes. *Diabetes.* 2006;55:1127–1132.

[24] Steppan J, Hofer S, Funke B et al. Sepsis and major abdominal surgery lead to flaking of the endothelial glycocalyx. *J Surg Res.* 2011;165:136–141.

[25] Johansson PI, Stensballe J, Rasmussen LS, Ostrowski SR. A high admission syndecan-1 level, a marker of endothelial glycocalyx degradation, is associated with inflammation, protein C depletion, fibrinolysis, and increased mortality in trauma patients. *Ann Surg.* 2011;254:194–200.

[26] Darnis E, Boysen S, et al. Establishment of reference values of the caudal vena cava by fast- ultrasonography through different views in healthy dogs. *J Vet Intern Med.* 2018;32:1308–1318.

[27] Oricco S, Rabozzi R, Meneghini C, Franci P. Usefulness of focused cardiac ultrasonography for predicting fluid responsiveness in conscious, spontaneously breathing dogs. *Am J Vet Res.* 2019;80:369–377.

[28] Sasaki K, Mutoh T et al. Electrical velocimetry for noninvasive cardiac output and stroke volume variation measurements in dogs undergoing cardiovascular surgery. *Vet Anaesth Analg.* 2017 Jan;44(1):7–16.

Clinical Case

Dehydrated dog with respiratory alkalosis

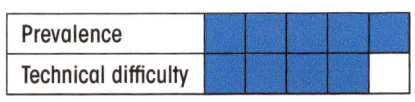

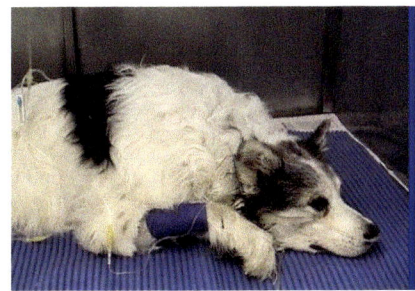

Signalment	
Name	Bianco
Species	canine
Breed	mixed breed
Sex	male
Weight	22 kg
Age	4 years

History

The patient was brought to the clinic because he had not been eating since the morning. He was able to drink, but occasionally regurgitated. His feces were normal, but more solid than usual. These clinical signs had been evident for at least 5 hours. The clinical parameters below were recorded during the clinical examination:
- Heart rate: 130 bpm;
- Respiratory rate: 40 bpm;
- Full pulse;
- Rectal temperature: 37.9 °C;
- mucous membranes: pinkish; CRT: 2 seconds;
- arterial pressure: 120/60 mmHg; MAP: 40 mmHg;
- dehydration: 8%.

Laboratory tests

A blood gas analysis was performed since the patient had been suffering from regurgitation and was likely to suffer from electrolytic and acid-base imbalances.

Chapter 1 ◆ Fundamentals of Fluid Therapy and Hemodynamics

Fluid therapy must be aimed at satisfying the patients' needs, so a complete blood count was performed to assess hematological parameters, as well as a biochemistry profile to evaluate a potential dysfunction of the organs related to the digestive system and check whether other metabolic components were also involved.

Venous blood gas analysis

Since there were no issues with the respiratory system, blood samples were taken from a vein given that these are reliable with regards to pH and bicarbonate, carbon dioxide and electrolyte levels:
- pH: 7.60;
- $pvCO_2$: 25;
- HCO_3^-: 24;
- BE: +5;
- Na^+: 135 mmol/L;
- Cl^-: 95 mmol/L;
- K^+: 3.2 mmol/L;
- lactatemia: 2.2 mmol/L;
- AG: 19.2;
- FiO_2: 0.21.

Biochemistry profile

BUN 15 mg/dL, creatinine 1.2 mg/dL, ALT 24 U/L, AST 31 U/L, total proteins 8.4 g/dL, albumin 5.3 g/dL, total bilirubin 0.2 mg/dL, GGT 12 U/L, blood glucose 104 mg/100 mL, phosphate 4.1 mg/dL.

Complete blood count

RBC 8.5×10^{12}/L, WBC 14.9×10^9/L, Hct 63%, Hb 16.3 g/dL, PLT 320×10^9/L, neutrophils 14×10^3/µL.

Interpretation of the results

The blood gas analysis showed evidence of respiratory alkalosis, since pCO_2 readings were low, while bicarbonate readings were normal. There was no evidence of bicarbonate compensation since it was too early for renal compensation to have kicked in in an attempt to withhold bicarbonate. The patient was therefore suffering from respiratory alkalosis, which had started a few hours earlier.

According to the nontraditional approach, a moderate alkalosis and SID alkalosis (−5 nmol/L) were present. In addition, a weak acid acidosis (increase in total proteins and albumin) was observed, which concealed and compensated for the respiratory alkalosis. Mild hypokalemia was also detected. The biochemistry profile highlighted an increase in total proteins and albumin, probably due to dehydration. The complete blood count showed an increased hematocrit, also probably due to dehydration. Osmolarity is calculated as follows:

$$Osm = 2 \times [Na+] + glucose (mg/dL)/18 + BUN (mg/dL)/2.8$$

$$Osm = (2 \times 135) + (104/18) + (15/2.8)$$

$$Osm = 281 \; mOsm/L$$

Osmolarity was lower than average due to hyponatremia.

Diagnostic investigations

An X-ray of the abdomen highlighted the presence of foreign objects in the patient's stomach, most probably stones, as shown in the picture.

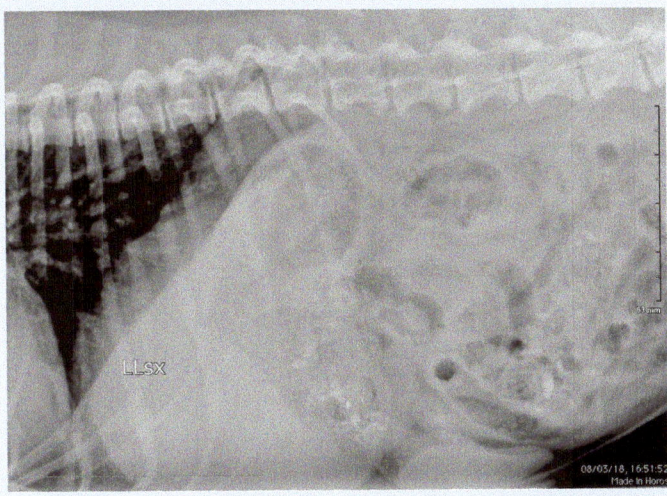

Chapter 1 ♦ Fundamentals of Fluid Therapy and Hemodynamics

Daily fluid therapy

Maintenance fluid therapy was provided, to which the volume corresponding to the percentage of dehydration (about 8%) was added, as well as the losses since the patient's arrival at the clinic (the dog had regurgitated 4 times, 30 mL each time). Resuscitative fluid therapy was not necessary since the patient was not showing signs of shock.

Ongoing: 2 mL/kg/hour IV, which corresponds to 44 mL/hour.

Rehydration: 8% of 22 kg corresponds to 1760 mL which, over 24 hours, corresponds to about 73 mL/hour EV.

This means that the total amount of solution to be administered for a least 24 hours was 117 mL/hour IV. In this case, 0.9% NaCl was chosen to restore the water and sodium lost due to regurgitation. Moreover, since normal saline is acid and it contains large amount of chloride, it is useful to normalize the water and electrolyte balance. There is no potassium in the solution, and it must therefore be added (see Chapter 4, Table 4.1). In this case, 15 mEq/L in 500 mL of potassium chloride were added. To correctly administer the solution an infusion pump is recommended. The patient's weight should be checked twice a day, while the electrolytes and acid–base status should be checked at least once every 24 hours.

The patient was treated this way for 24 hours; then the 76 mL/hour of the rehydration solution were subtracted from the total volume.

The patient was discharged the following day since regurgitation had stopped and he was eating and drinking spontaneously. Since the foreign objects were very small, they did not pose a threat to the transit of food through the digestive tract. The at-home supportive treatment included a mild proton pump inhibitor for 7 days (pantoprazole 1 mg/kg twice a day PO) and an intestinal absorbent (diosmectite 1 g twice a day PO for 7 days) to promote recovery from the possible lesions the foreign objects could have caused to the gastrointestinal mucosa.

Acid–Base Disorders

Fabio Viganò

CHAPTER 2

Introduction

When fluid therapy is required, it is important to know, in addition to the electrolyte status, the acid–base balance of the patient. In this chapter, acid–base disturbances will first be evaluated based on the traditional approach, before being analyzed according to a nontraditional approach (the Stewart approach), for a better understanding of how some electrolytes and ions can influence the acid–base balance.

One interpretation, however, does not exclude the other; indeed, both complement each other to provide an overview that allows an evaluation of the greatest number of components of the acid–base balance.

Chemical species involved in the acid–base balance

Under normal conditions, the body produces more acidic chemical species (about 15,000–20,000 mEq) than buffer systems (about 2500 mEq); it must therefore be able to quickly eliminate or buffer excess acids.

The body has a better ability to correct acidosis than alkalosis, and thus tolerates metabolic acidosis better than metabolic alkalosis.

A dog running in a field during a walk may have some degree of metabolic acidosis, but this will be corrected promptly; however, if the effort, because of its intensity and duration, were to exceed the normal compensation capacity, acidosis could become incompatible with life or create acid–base disorders with a negative impact on several of the animal's vital functions.

It is the clinician's task to identify as early as possible severe uncompensated acid–base alterations that could compromise the patient's vital functions.

Carbon dioxide (CO_2) acts as an acid in the body because carbonic anhydrase, a ubiquitous enzyme, catalyzes a reaction that converts CO_2 and water into carbonic acid (H_2CO_3). With an increase in partial pressure of carbon dioxide ($PaCO_2$),

Chapter 2 ◆ Acid–Base Disorders

the carbonic acid equation (Equation 1) will shift to the right and the hydrogen ion concentration will increase:

$$CO_2 + H_2O \leftrightarrow H_2CO_3 \leftrightarrow H_2^+ + HCO_3^- \qquad (Equation\ 1)$$

CO_2, in addition to being transformed into H_2CO_3, is mainly eliminated through alveolar ventilation. If alveolar ventilation is compromised (e.g., due to pneumothorax or positive pressure ventilation with high levels of CO_2), this mechanism becomes ineffective and the reaction will shift to the right. Alveolar ventilation can change the CO_2 concentration within 1–5 minutes; for example, if a patient has an increased respiratory rate as a result of fear or pain during blood sampling, the blood gas analysis (ABG) may indicate a false respiratory alkalosis (decreased CO_2).

While the respiratory system can correct the pH through alveolar ventilation within a few minutes, renal adaptation, which is characterized by bicarbonate reabsorption (80–90% of which occurs in the proximal tubule) and excretion of ammonium and phosphate ions and water, needs a few hours to begin and is completed within 2–5 days.

According to the law of mass action, the elements of the chemical species indicated in Equation 1 (Box 2.1) must remain in equilibrium on both sides of the equation. For example, if HCO_3^- increases, as occurs when sodium bicarbonate is administered, the reaction will tend to shift to the left; but if the patient's ventilation is impaired, the reaction will shift to the right, thus inducing a paradoxical acidosis. That is why the patient's ventilation should be assessed before administering sodium bicarbonate.

Similarly, when the equilibrium shifts to the right with an increase in H⁺ ions, it must be compensated for by a greater production of HCO_3^- by the kidneys since the HCO_3^- generated by the reaction is consumed by fixed acids. As a result, when kidney function is compromised, metabolic acidosis occurs.

It may be more useful to use the Stewart approach for proper fluid therapy; in patients with mixed or complex acid–base disorders, this approach also provides a

Box 2.1	Chemical species involved in acid–base disorders, traditional approach
• CO_2 • H^+ • HCO_3^- • H_2O	

Chapter 2 ◆ Acid–Base Disorders

more comprehensive evaluation of the acid–base status and a greater insight into its possible causes and the most appropriate treatment. However, before describing the Stewart approach, the traditional acid–base analysis will be discussed.

Traditional approach

The traditional approach is based on the Henderson–Hasselbalch equation (Equation 2) and considers bicarbonate concentration (HCO_3^-) and partial pressure of carbonic dioxide (PCO_2). The formula uses the common logarithm of the molar concentration of hydrogen ions, which would otherwise generate complex numbers: 0.0000001 gEq/L or 1×10^{-7} H^+.

$$pH = 6.1 + \log \frac{[HCO_3^-]}{0.03 \times PCO_2} \qquad (Equation\ 2)$$

From this equation, it can easily be seen that an increase in HCO_3^- concentration will be responsible for an increase in pH (alkalosis), while a decrease will cause the opposite phenomenon. Conversely, an increased CO_2 concentration will be responsible for a decreased pH (acidosis), whereas a drop in CO_2 concentration will cause an increase in pH. Because they are retained by the kidneys, HCO_3^- ions are defined as a metabolic component of the acid–base balance, while CO_2, which is primarily removed by alveolar ventilation, is defined as a respiratory component. A $PaCO_2$ greater than 45 mmHg is termed respiratory acidosis, while a $PaCO_2$ below 35 mmHg defines respiratory alkalosis. Metabolic acidosis, on the other hand, occurs when HCO_3^- falls below 20 and metabolic alkalosis when it is greater than 24.

An increase in H^+ ions in blood results in acidemia, i.e., a decreased pH (<7.35); conversely, a decrease in H^+ ions in blood results in alkalemia, i.e., an increased pH (>7.45). The suffix "-emia" indicates the presence of a certain kind of substance in the blood that causes an imbalance, while the suffix "-osis" (acidosis or alkalosis) indicates the development of a condition (Box 2.2).

If the fixed acids produced by the body are not eliminated or buffered, metabolic acidosis occurs. Some of them are eliminated by alveolar ventilation, such as CO_2 and water; this process begins within a few minutes and is completed within a few hours. An acid can be buffered or excreted through metabolic pathways. It can be buffered by bicarbonate (in the renal proximal tubules, 40% of the total buffering capacity), by hemoglobin (35% of the buffer system and 80% of the nonbicarbonate buffer system), by the formation of ammonium ions (NH_4^+, in the renal col-

Chapter 2 ◆ Acid–Base Disorders

Box 2.2	Effects of chemical species on pH, traditional approach

- An increase in H⁺ ions causes a reduction in pH.
- A reduction in H⁺ ions causes an increase in pH.
- An increase in CO_2 causes a reduction in pH.
- A reduction in CO_2 causes an increase in pH.
- An increase in HCO_3^- causes an increase in pH.
- A reduction in HCO_3^- causes a reduction in pH.

lecting tubule), by proteins (which represent 7% of the buffer system and of which albumin is the most abundant), by ATP (adenosine triphosphate), by 2,3-diphosphoglycerate, and by organic (3% of buffer system) and inorganic (2% of buffer system) phosphates.

Blood gas analyzers

Blood gas analyzers measure pH, PCO_2 and PaO_2 and calculate bicarbonate and base excess (BE). The conversion factor from mmHg to kPa is 0.133 and 7.5006 from KPa to mmHg. Devices with a cooxymeter can also measure the percentage of saturation of hemoglobin, the percentage of carboxyhemoglobin, the percentage of methemoglobin and the amount of hemoglobin. Most modern blood gas analyzers also measure electrolytes such as sodium, potassium, chloride and calcium, and some of them determine blood lactate and glucose concentrations, urea, creatinine, cardiac troponin, activated coagulation time and total bilirubin.

The determination of electrolytes, along with the measurement of total proteins, albumin, and phosphates (with other instruments), also allows an interpretation of acid–base disorders using the Stewart approach. The equipment should also measure electrolytes to help the clinician select the appropriate fluid therapy, correct electrolyte imbalances, and monitor the speed of correction of these imbalances. Not all devices use the same algorithms to calculate values, so it is advisable to always ask the supplier about the mathematical formulas used for the determination of BE and bicarbonate, and whether the device distinguishes between the canine and feline species (Table 2.1).

Chapter 2 ◆ Acid–Base Disorders

Table 2.1 Normal values of blood gas analysis in dogs and cats

Parameter	Dog A	Dog AR	Dog V	Dog VR	Cat A	Cat AR	Cat V	Cat VR
pH	7.4	7.35–7.45	7.40	7.32–7.50	7.39	7.24–7.45	7.36	7.28–7.41
CO_2	38	35–45	35.3	33–50	37	25–37	40.8	33–45
HCO_3^-	24	22–27	22.3	18–26	18	15–22	22.4	18–23
O_2	92	80–110			107	96–118	39.1	35–45
BE	±2	−2–+2	±2	−2–+2	±2.5	−2–+2.5	+2.5	−2–+2.5
AG		12–20		12–20	12–18	12–18		12–18
TCO_2		23–29		23–29	15–20	15–20		15–20
SpO_2	>90				<85			
A–a	10–20				10–20			

A, arterial; AR, arterial range; V, venous; VR, venous range.
A–a, alveolar–arterial gradient; AG, anion gap; BE, base excess; CO_2, carbon dioxide; HCO_3^-, bicarbonate; O_2, oxygen; pH, concentration of hydrogen ions; SpO_2, percentage of oxygen-saturated hemoglobin; TCO_2, total carbon dioxide.

Chapter 2 ◆ Acid–Base Disorders

Interpretation of blood gas analysis

Primary disorder

Once the arterial blood gas (ABG) has been performed, the clinician must identify the primary disorder, that is, understand whether the metabolic or respiratory component varies in the same direction as pH. For example, if the pH value is acidic, it must be determined if it is the respiratory component (CO_2) that produces the acidosis (after an increase in CO_2 concentration), or if it is the metabolic component that that lowers the pH (with a reduction in HCO_3^-). The reading sequence of a blood gas analysis should be as follows:
- pH;
- CO_2;
- HCO_3^-.

The identification of the primary disorder is fundamental to treat its origin because the adaptive response depends on it, but not only for that reason: if at least two separate primary acid–base disturbances are present simultaneously, treating the main one will often correct the entire acid–base imbalance. Some examples are given below.

The first parameter that should be assessed is therefore pH, which should then be compared with normal values (acidosis or alkalosis, see Table 2.1). This should be followed by evaluation of the PCO_2: if it is altered in the same direction as pH, a respiratory disorder is in progress. For example, if pH is <7.35 and the PCO_2 is >45–50 mmHg, the primary disorder is respiratory acidosis; conversely, if the pH is >7.35 and the PCO_2 is <40 mmHg the primary disorder is respiratory alkalosis. The clinician should then look at the HCO_3^- concentration: if the PCO_2 is normal while HCO_3^- goes in the same direction as the pH alteration, the disorder has a metabolic origin. For example, if the pH is >7.45, the PCO_2 is normal, and HCO_3^- is >24, the primary disorder is a metabolic alkalosis; conversely, if the pH is <7.4, the PCO_2 is normal, and HCO_3^- is <20 mEq/L, the patient is suffering from a metabolic acidosis. Once the primary disorder has been identified, it is necessary to check whether the clinical findings are concordant with the ABG values. For example, if a respiratory alkalosis is diagnosed, the respiratory pattern and rate should be assessed and, if necessary, additional tests performed (e.g., diagnostic imaging) (Box 2.3).

Compensatory responses

When an acid–base imbalance (acidosis or alkalosis) occurs, the body responds with a compensatory mechanism. For example, in respiratory acidosis, the opposite reac-

Chapter 2 ◆ Acid–Base Disorders

> **Box 2.3** — **Primary disorder, traditional approach**
>
> - If the pH decreases and CO_2 increases, respiratory acidosis is the primary disorder.
> - If the pH increases and CO_2 decreases, respiratory alkalosis is the primary disorder.
> - If the pH decreases and HCO_3^- decreases, metabolic acidosis is the primary disorder.
> - If the pH increases and HCO_3^- increases, metabolic alkalosis is the primary disorder.

tion to compensate for the alteration in pH will be a metabolic alkalosis. The type of compensatory response depends on the acid–base imbalance and on when it is established (Table 2.2).

It should be remembered that the body never overcompensates. This means that the increase or reduction in the $PaCO_2$ and HCO_3^- beyond the compensation values indicated in Table 2.2 are suggestive of the presence of another pathological condition; these are defined as mixed acid–base disorders. There are no guidelines regarding compensatory responses in cats, and the values for dogs generally serve as a reference, although their accuracy in the feline species has not been established, especially with regard to respiratory compensation.

Table 2.3 shows some characteristic examples of acid–base disturbances.

Table 2.2 Normal compensation

Primary disorder	Alteration	Compensatory response
Metabolic acidosis	HCO_3^- reduction of 1 mEq/L	$PaCO_2$ reduction of 0.7 mmHg
Metabolic alkalosis	HCO_3^- increase of 1 mEq/L	$PaCO_2$ increase of 0.7 mmHg
Respiratory acidosis Acute Chronic	 $PaCO_2$ increase of 1 mmHg $PaCO_2$ increase of 1 mmHg	 HCO_3^- increase of 0.15 mEq/L HCO_3^- increase of 0.35 mEq/L
Respiratory alkalosis Acute Chronic	 $PaCO_2$ reduction of 1 mmHg $PaCO_2$ reduction of 1 mmHg	 HCO_3^- reduction of 0.25 mEq/L HCO_3^- reduction of 0.55 mEq/L

HCO_3^-, bicarbonate ion concentration; $paCO_2$, partial pressure of carbon dioxide.

Chapter 2 ◆ Acid–Base Disorders

Table 2.3 Examples of diseases associated with acid-base disorders

Imbalance	Diseases
Respiratory acidosis	Diseases of pleural space, anesthetic drugs, airway obstruction, compensation of metabolic alkalosis, parenteral feeding with excess carbohydrates, central nervous system diseases, ineffective positive pressure ventilation
Metabolic acidosis	Normal anion gap: diarrhea, proximal tubular acidosis (inability to tubular reabsorption), compensation of respiratory alkalosis, dilution acidosis (excessive administration of 0.9% saline solution), hypoadrenocorticism, carbonic anhydrase inhibitor, administration of ammonium chloride, parenteral nutrition with cationic amino acids (e.g., lysine, arginine, histidine) High anion gap: lactic acidosis, diabetic ketoacidosis, hyperphosphatemia, phosphate and sulfate acidosis (oliguric renal failure), salicylate intoxication, ethylene glycol intoxication, metaldehyde intoxication, paraldehyde intoxication, methanol intoxication, severe rhabdomyolysis
Respiratory alkalosis	Hyperventilation (e.g., pain), restrictive respiratory distress, hypotension, anxiety, exercise, compensation for metabolic acidosis, congestive heart failure
Metabolic alkalosis	Vomiting, hypokalemia, refeeding after fasting, loss of renal function due thiazides, mineralocorticoids, high doses of β-lactam antibiotics, hypovolemic alkalosis, compensation of respiratory acidosis, posthypercapnia, administration of bicarbonate, fluid therapy with alkalizing solutions

In many cases it is possible to find simultaneous metabolic and respiratory alterations in opposite directions; the resulting pH can be normal or almost normal, and such alterations are called mixed acid–base disorders. Mixed acid–base disorders do not always go in the opposite direction; two or more pathological conditions in the same patient can all induce acidosis or alkalosis. These pathological alterations are the most difficult to diagnose and manage because, if they are not readily recognized and treated, they can quickly lead to a fatal outcome. To determine which of the disturbances should be treated first, it is necessary to perform another evaluation of the patient's clinical condition; for example, if a patient has a metabolic acidosis due to severe diarrhea and a respiratory acidosis resulting from a severe central nervous system (CNS) depression (e.g., stupor or coma), we must first treat the disease that most impairs the animal's vital functions.

Chapter 2 ◆ Acid–Base Disorders

An ABG should be performed not only when acid–base imbalances exist or are suspected, or when fluid therapy is to be performed, but also in all patients with disturbances in the extracellular space (e.g., dehydration, vomiting, diarrhea and hypovolemia) or electrolytes, in those with respiratory or cardiorespiratory diseases requiring general anesthesia, and in all critically ill patients suffering from any pathological processes that may compromise their vital functions.

Base excess (BE)

BE is part of the buffer system, which includes not only the bicarbonate system but also hemoglobin. The BE indicates the amount of strong base or acid that must be added to 1 L of oxygenated whole blood to restore the pH to 7.4 at 37 °C and at a $PaCO_2$ of 40 mmHg. A normal value of BE is about 0 (±2). In cats it is slightly lower and influenced only by the amount of fixed acids; it is therefore an indicator of the metabolic state. A reduced BE indicates metabolic acidosis, while an increased BE indicates metabolic alkalosis.

An altered BE value may be normal and may indicate the body's compensatory response. For example, a patient with chronic respiratory acidosis (e.g., secondary to an obstructive pulmonary disease) may have a BE above normal to buffer a chronic increase in CO_2 and therefore in the H^+ ions present in the blood; in this case, a high BE is not a pathological finding, but rather indicates an adaptive response to a chronic acid–base disorder. An increased BE may be due to an increase in bases or a decrease in fixed acids; a decreased BE may be due to a decrease in bases or an increase in fixed acids. BE is especially useful during metabolic acidosis to confirm and understand if the disorder is compensated for by bases or if it is necessary to intervene with appropriate therapy. In the latter case, if the BE is below normal, the clinician must decide whether the disorder should be corrected by administering buffer systems (nonbicarbonate buffer or bicarbonate) or by limiting the production of acid.

Anion gap (AG)

When reading an ABG and diagnosing metabolic acidosis, it is important to read the AG value. In the body, electroneutrality between all ions must be maintained, so there must be an equal number of cations and anions in the blood; however, not all cations and anions are normally measured.

Measured cations are more than measured anions, so the difference will be in favor of cations, which is why this is referred to as the AG (see Equation 5). In other words, there are more unmeasured anions (UAs) than unmeasured cations (UCs) and the AG has a positive value. The commonly measured cations are sodium (Na^+) and potassium (K^+), while the commonly measured anions are chloride (Cl^-) and

Chapter 2 ♦ Acid–Base Disorders

bicarbonate (HCO_3^-). The most frequently unmeasured cations are calcium (Ca^{2+}) and magnesium (Mg^{2+}), while unmeasured anions are proteins, of which albumin is the most abundant, and lactate, phosphates and sulfates.

The balance between cations and anions is summarized by the following equations:

$$(Na^+ + K^+) + UCs^+ = (Cl^- + HCO_3^-) + UAs^- \qquad (Equation\ 3)$$

The difference between cations and anions is calculated using the terms from the previous equation:

$$AG = [(Na^+ + K^+) + UCs^+] - [(Cl^- + HCO_3^-) + UAs^-] \qquad (Equation\ 4)$$

Simplifying the formula, the AG is calculated by subtracting the measured anions from the measured cations:

$$AG = (Na^+ + K^+) - (Cl^- + HCO_3^-) \qquad (Equation\ 5)$$

The normal AG value is approximately 12 to 20 mmol/L. When UAs increase, major anions ($Cl^- + HCO_3^-$) must decrease to maintain an electrolyte balance, which causes an increase in the AG. Some diseases increase the presence of fixed acids with negative charges, which become part of the UAs responsible for metabolic acidosis and an *increased AG*, such as:
- lactic acidosis;
- diabetic ketoacidosis;
- renal failure (uremia and increased phosphates and sulfates);
- rhabdomyolysis;
- sepsis;
- convulsion;
- poisonings: ethylene glycol, methylene glycol, alcohol, salicylates, paraldehyde, iron.

These pathological processes, also referred to as normochloremic or hypochloremic metabolic acidosis, are characterized by an increase in UAs (e.g., lactate and ketones), and chloride ions must decrease accordingly or remain normal to compensate for the increase in negative electrical charges (UAs).

Metabolic acidosis with an *increased AG* is typical of renal failure and diarrhea. In response to bicarbonate losses resulting from diarrhea, a compensatory retention of chloride ions occurs to maintain electroneutrality. This type of acidosis is therefore called hyperchloremic metabolic acidosis.

Chapter 2 ◆ Acid–Base Disorders

Box 2.4	Metabolic acidosis and anion gap
Increased anion gap • Lactic acidosis • Ketoacidosis • Renal failure: uremia and increased phosphates and sulfates • Sepsis • Seizures • Poisonings: ethylene glycol, methylene glycol, alcohol, salicylates, paraldehyde, iron • Rhabdomyolysis	**Normal anion gap** • Diarrhea, duodenal vomiting • Renal tubular acidosis • Administration of NaCl • Compensation of respiratory alkalosis • Parenteral nutrition (increased amino acids: arginine, lysine, histidine, cystine, methionine) • Hypoadrenocorticism • Ammonium chloride or acetazolamide therapy

Therefore, in the course of metabolic acidosis, chloride ions can increase to compensate for a reduction in bicarbonate or decrease as UAs increase.

In conclusion, the AG is useful to better define the origin of metabolic acidosis. When diagnosing metabolic acidosis, it is thus necessary to check if the AG is normal or increased. When it is increased or normal, the list of differential diagnoses should be examined to identify the possible cause (Box 2.4).

Total oxygen content (CaO_2)

CaO_2 is the total amount of oxygen present in the blood. Part of the oxygen is bound to hemoglobin (component in greater amount) and a small amount is dissolved in blood. The amount of dissolved oxygen is proportional to the partial pressure of oxygen and its solubility coefficient. Oxygen has a plasma solubility of 0.003 and each gram of hemoglobin saturated with 100% of oxygen carries 1.34 mL of oxygen, so CaO_2 is calculated using the following formula:

$$CaO_2 = (PaO_2 \times 0.003) + (1.34 \times Hb \times SaO_2) \qquad (Equation\ 6)$$

As can be seen in the formula, most of the oxygen contained in the blood is bound to hemoglobin, while the oxygen dissolved by the pressure gradient ($PaO_2 \times 0.003$) represents only a small part of the total. For example, if a patient has a hemoglobin saturation (SaO$_2$) of 98%, a PaO$_2$ of 95 mmHg, and 10 g/dL of hemoglobin, the CaO$_2$ can be calculated as follows:

$$CaO_2 = (95 \times 0.003) + (1.34 \times 10 \times 0.98) \qquad (Equation\ 7)$$

$$13{,}417 = (0.285) + (13.132) \qquad (Equation\ 8)$$

Using this calculation, it is possible to assess the magnitude of the decrease in blood oxygen content if a patient suffers an acute hemorrhage causing the loss of half of their hemoglobin. The CaO$_2$ would be reduced by about half, thus decreasing drastically the patient's chances of survival. This is because CaO$_2$ and cardiac output (CO) constitute the two fundamental components of oxygen availability (DO$_2$), according to the following calculation: $(95 \times 0.003) + (1.34 \times 5 \times 0.98) = 6.851$.

If oxygen is administered to this patient, for example through a nasal cannula, the percentage of inhaled oxygen will become about 40%, which will increase the PaO$_2$ from about 95 to 200 mmHg. The CaO$_2$, however, will only increase slightly (comparing it with the normal value, Equation 7), according to the following calculation: $(200 \times 0.003) + (1.34 \times 5 \times 0.98) = 7.166$.

In anemic patients, hemoglobin should be administered (e.g., using packed red blood cells) to significantly increase the CaO$_2$ and consequently the chances of survival. If only the fraction of inspired oxygen (FiO$_2$) is increased by administering oxygen, a significant increase in CaO$_2$ will not be achieved; despite this, in some patients, even a modest increase in CaO$_2$ achieved through oxygen therapy can favor a positive outcome. As it is impossible to know in advance which anemic patients can survive thanks to oxygen therapy, it is a good idea to always administer oxygen in these critically ill patients.

Oxygen parameters to evaluate the effectiveness of oxygenation

By measuring the alveolar–arterial gradient (A–a) or the PaO$_2$/FiO$_2$ ratio, it is possible to determine the amount of oxygenated blood and quantify the shunt fraction, that is, the amount of blood that travels through the lungs without receiving oxygenation. The most common causes of pulmonary shunts are post-traumatic pulmonary insufficiency, pulmonary edema, acute respiratory distress syndrome (ARDS), pulmonary atelectasis (e.g., as a result of prolonged decubitus), aspiration pneumonia, some lung neoplasms, inhalation of toxic gases, some bronchospastic diseases (e.g., asthma, alveolar lung diseases, and bronchospasm), and, finally, right-to-left anatomic shunts (e.g., patent ductus arteriosus, tetralogy of Fallot and atrioventricular fistula).

Chapter 2 ◆ Acid–Base Disorders

Alveolar–arterial gradient

The **alveolar–arterial gradient** (A–a gradient) is calculated by measuring the difference between the oxygen present in the pulmonary alveoli (pAO_2) and the oxygen is present in the blood (PaO_2). It is an index of the ability of the cardiovascular and respiratory systems to transfer oxygen from room air to the blood. The alveolar–arterial gradient is the difference between the calculated alveolar partial pressure of oxygen and the measured arterial partial pressure of oxygen:

$$A\text{–}a = pAO_2 - PaO_2 \qquad (Equation\ 9)$$

$$pAO_2 = FiO_2 \times (\text{barometric pressure} - 47) - (PaCO_2/0.8) \qquad (Equation\ 10)$$

In the first part of the Equation 10, the partial pressure of oxygen in room air is measured by multiplying the FiO_2 (fraction of inspired oxygen) by the barometric pressure subtracted from the partial pressure of water vapor (barometric pressure – 47); in the second part of the equation, the ratio between the $PaCO_2$ (partial pressure of carbon dioxide) and R (respiratory quotient, 0.8) must be subtracted from the amount of oxygen obtained from the first part of the equation.

In healthy patients, with an FiO_2 of 0.21 because they breathe room air, the A–a gradient should be less than or equal to 15 mmHg; higher values indicate a deficit in the ventilation/perfusion ratio (V/Q). Over the course of parenchymal lung diseases (e.g., pneumonia, ARDS, post-traumatic pulmonary insufficiency), the V/Q ratio increases and is the cause of hypoxemia. The higher the V/Q ratio, the greater the hypoxemia. The difference between the oxygen present in the alveoli and that present in the arterial blood is due to impaired oxygen diffusion through the lung parenchyma and is not necessarily affected by the inhaled oxygen. The A–a gradient also increases in cases of diffusion hypoxia and right-to-left pulmonary shunts. Therefore, the A–a gradient is important to understand the severity of some lung diseases, establish therapy (e.g., need for oxygen therapy or positive pressure ventilation), assess the course of the disease process, and monitor the effectiveness of therapy. When, despite oxygen therapy, no improvement in the A–a gradient is achieved, the need for positive pressure ventilation should be considered. The greater the measured value, the more severe the oxygen deficit. Values between 10 and 20 indicate a slight deficit, values greater than 30 indicate severely impaired oxygen diffusion.

PaO_2/FiO_2 ratio

Another method to assess the body's ability to oxygenate the blood is to measure the partial pressure of oxygen in arterial blood and divide it by the fraction of inspired oxygen: **PaO_2/FiO_2**. This is the most frequently used method to evaluate the oxygenation capacity because it is very simple and the ratio can be calculated even when patients are undergoing oxygen therapy, considering FiO_2 is a value that can be set arbitrarily depending on the therapy that the patient is receiving. Therefore, for patients breathing room air it is possible to use the A–a gradient, while for patients on oxygen therapy the PaO_2/FiO_2 ratio must be used and the FiO_2 adjusted when necessary. Under normal conditions, the PaO_2/FiO_2 ratio should be greater than or equal to about 500 (105/0.21); values between 300 and 500 indicate mild hypoxemia, while values between 200 and 300 reveal moderate to severe hypoxemia (e.g., acute lung injury [ALI]), and values below 200 indicate severe hypoxemia (e.g., acute respiratory distress syndrome).

This method is used to differentiate, together with other clinical findings (e.g., presence of a pathology able to cause ARDS, chest X-rays, presence of high concentration of proteins in the surfactant, absence of heart disease), ALI from ARDS (<200) (Box 2.5). When it is necessary to assess the lungs' efficiency in oxygenating blood, especially during oxygen therapy, the PaO_2/FiO_2 ratio is the most frequently used method, because it is very simple, quick, and effective in assessing the severity of hypoxemia and in monitoring the effectiveness of treatment. This method can be used for normal atmospheric pressures (comparable to that of sea level). FiO_2 can be given as a percentage or fraction, with conversion of FiO_2 in L/min to a percentage value using the following equation:

$$FiO_2 \text{ L/min} = (FiO_2 \% - 21)/3 \qquad (Equation\ 11)$$

For example, the following values can be obtained: 1 L/min = 24%, 3 L/min = 30%, 5 L/min = 36%, 6 L/min = 39%.

Box 2.5 — **PaO_2/FiO_2 ratio, clinical interpretation**

- 500 = normal value
- 300–500 = mild hypoxemia
- 200–300 = moderate/severe hypoxemia (e.g., ALI)
- <200 = very serious hypoxemia (e.g., ARDS)

Chapter 2 ◆ Acid–Base Disorders

Rule of 5

A very practical and empirical method for assessing the ability to oxygenate the blood is the rule of 5. In practice, the FiO_2 is multiplied by 5, and the value obtained is compared with the PaO_2. For example, in a patient who breathes room air, the PaO_2 should be about 100 mmHg (21% × 5); if the patient receives oxygen through a nasal cannula, their PaO_2 should be about 200 mmHg (40% × 5). Values lower than expected indicate hypoxia. This method can be used for normal atmospheric pressures (comparable to that of sea level).

Rule of 120

The rule of 120, on the other hand, refers to the sum of the arterial partial pressures of oxygen and carbon dioxide. This sum normally should normally be between 120 and 160 mmHg; if it is less than 120 mmHg there is insufficient oxygen exchange at the alveolar level and the cause of the hypoxia must be investigated. This method can only be used if the patient breathes room air at normal atmospheric pressures (comparable to that of sea level).

Strong ion theory (Stewart's approach)

The strong ion theory was elaborated by Peter Stewart in 1983 and draws its foundations from the laws of mass action and electroneutrality. According to these physical laws, the quantity of chemical species involved in the acid–base balance remains constant until a certain amount is added, generated, removed or destroyed, while electroneutrality must be maintained (the sum of the positive charges must be equal to the sum of the negative charges).

The interpretation of acid–base imbalances according to the strong ion theory is very useful for fluid therapy, as it allows us to understand some of these imbalances especially with regard to electrolytes and fluid administration, but also when weak acids (A_{tot}) and phosphates are involved.

Chemical species involved

According to the laws of mass action and electroneutrality, if a positive or negative charge increases, H^+ or OH^- concentrations must change to balance the charge (e.g., if Cl^- increases, H^+ must increase to compensate for the alteration in the electric charge), thereby changing the pH. According to this approach, the only three

Chapter 2 ◆ Acid–Base Disorders

independent variables—i.e., those that can vary in quantity independently from each other—are:
- CO_2;
- A_{tot} (total weak acids);
- SID (strong ion difference).

CO_2, as in the traditional approach, is conditioned by ventilation (an increase in frequency causes a reduction in CO_2 and vice versa).

Nonvolatile A_{tot} (total weak acids) are proteins (under normal conditions, these make up 90% of A_{tot}), predominantly total proteins, albumin and inorganic phosphate.

The SID corresponds to the difference between strong ions, which depend on metabolism, imbalances in the extracellular space, and fluid therapy. The balance of the SID can be obtained by subtracting anions from cations, as shown in the following equation:

$$\text{SID} = \underbrace{(Na^+ + Ca^{2+} + Mg^{2+} + K^+)}_{\cong 150} - \underbrace{(Cl^- + PO_4^{2-} + Alb^- + \text{globulins} + KK + \text{lactate}^-)}_{\cong 118}$$

(Equation 12)

SID, strong ion difference; PO_4^{2-}, phosphates; Alb^-, albumin; KK, ketone bodies.

The SID is so called because, at pH 7.4, ions completely dissociate and are found dissolved in the blood practically only as positive or negative charges. The ions found in higher concentrations are Na^+ and Cl^- (Box 2.6). In the traditional approach the independent variables depend on renal and pulmonary function, perfusion and metabolism, while according to the Stewart approach, the independent variables also depend on liver function (Figure 2.1).

Box 2.6 — **Chemical species involved in acid–base disturbances, nontraditional approach**

- CO_2.
- A_{tot} (total weak acids): total proteins, albumin, phosphates.
- Strong ions: Na^+, Ca^{2+}, Mg^{2+}, Cl^-, PO_4^{2-}, lactate, ketone bodies.
- With an increase in positive charge, H^+ must be reduced; with an increase in the negative charges, H^+ must increase.
- Reductions in SID cause metabolic acidosis.

Chapter 2 ◆ Acid–Base Disorders

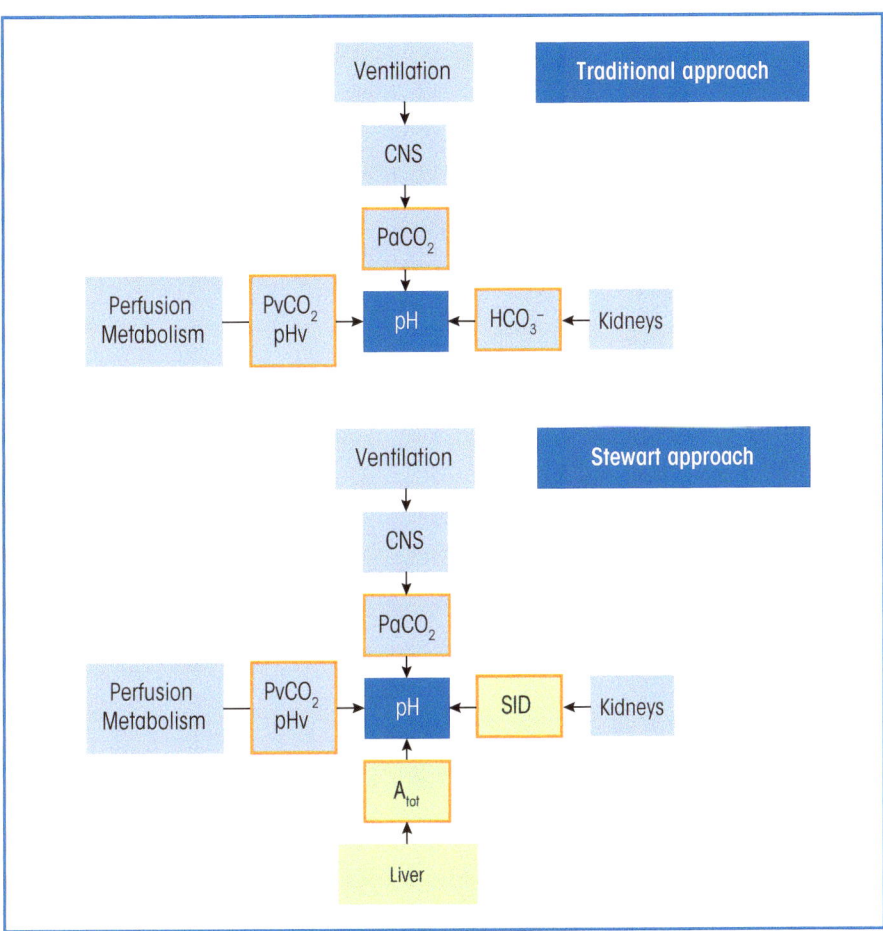

Figure 2.1 Comparison between the components of the traditional approach and Stewart approach.

Tables 2.4 and 2.5 show the contribution to the acid–base equilibrium of sodium, chloride, water and A_{tot}. Alterations in concentrations of strong cations or strong anions are responsible for acid–base alterations. If you want evaluate pH using the Stewart approach by modifying the Henderson–Hasselbalch equation, the components that influence pH are:

$$pH = \frac{6.1 + (SID - A_{tot})}{(0.03 \times PCO_2)} \qquad (Equation\ 13)$$

Independent variables are indicated in blue, while dependent variables in black.

Chapter 2 ♦ Acid–Base Disorders

Table 2.4 Biological behavior of various components of the acid-base disorders according to the nontraditional approach

Component	Consequence
↓ Water ⇒ ↑ [Na^+] ⇒ ↓ [H_+]	Hypovolemic alkalosis
↑ Water ⇒ ↓ [Na^+] ⇒ ↑ [H_+]	Hypervolemic acidosis
↑ [Cl^-] ⇒ ↑ [H^+] ⇒ ↓ pH	Hyperchloremic acidosis
↓ [Cl^-] ⇒ ↓ [H^+] ⇒ ↑ pH	Hypochloremic alkalosis
↑ [Pr^-] ⇒ ↑ [H^+] ⇒ ↓ pH	High-protein acidosis
↓ [Pr^-] ⇒ ↓ [H^+] ⇒ ↑ pH	Low-protein alkalosis
↓ [$Albumin^-$] ⇒ ↓ [H^+] ⇒ ↑ pH	Hypoalbuminemic alkalosis
↑ [$Albumin^-$] ⇒ ↑ [H^+] ⇒ ↓ pH	High-protein acidosis
↑ [$Cations^+$] ⇒ ↓ [H^+]	Alkalizing effect
↑ [$Lactate^-$] ⇒ ↑ [H^+] ⇒ ↓ pH	Acidifying effect
↑ [UAs^-] ⇒ ↑ [H^+] ⇒ ↓ pH	Acidifying effect

Table 2.5 Calculation of the effect of strong ions on the base excess

Na^+	0.25 × (Na^+ patient – 145) dog 0.22 × (Na^+ patient – 155) cat
Cl^-	110 – (Cl^- × 145/Na^+) dog 120 – (Cl^- × 155/Na^+) cat
Contribution from proteins or contribution from albumin	3 × (6.5 – TP) or 3.7 × (3.1 – albumin)
Phosphates	0.58 × (normal phosphate mg/dL – patient phosphates mg/dL)
Lactate	–1 × [lactate]
Effect of unmeasured anions	UAs = BE – (Na^+ + Cl^- + Pr^- o Alb^- + lactate)

BE, base excess calculated with blood gas analysis; UAs, unmeasured anions.

Chapter 2 ◆ Acid–Base Disorders

Box 2.7	Features of the nontraditional approach

- An increase in positive charges induces a reduction in H⁺ (alkalosis).
- An increase in negative charges induces an increase in H⁺ (acidosis).
- An increase in SID causes a reduction in H⁺ and thus induces alkalosis.
- A reduction in SID causes an increase in H⁺ and thus induces acidosis.
- The SID can change, in general, due to variations in the water volumes (sodium), chloride, strong negative ions (albumin, lactate, phosphates, ketone bodies, globulins).

Dependent and independent variables

According to the traditional approach (see Equation 2), the dependent variable is H⁺, while the independent variables are $PaCO_2$ and HCO_3^-; according to the nontraditional approach, however, the dependent variables are H⁺ and HCO_3^-, while the independent variables are $PaCO_2$, SID and A_{tot}. In other words, it can be said that the pH is conditioned by variations in CO_2, SID and A_{tot}; for this reason, when analyzing a clinical case, if these last three elements are within the reference range, the traditional approach is sufficient to understand the possible acid–base disturbance.

Each component of the nontraditional approach has a different influence, which can be described as in Table 2.4. Looking at Table 2.5, it can easily be inferred that the greatest influence on pH is produced by a reduction in SID. A reduction in UAs, produced by the difference between the BE and the contribution of all strong ions, indicates the presence of unmeasured strong anions (UAs) or cations responsible for acid–base disturbances (Box 2.7).

Examples of pH variations according to the nontraditional approach

Pure water losses cause an increase in Na⁺ concentration, which has an alkalizing effect because the number of cations is increased and the number of H⁺ ions must decrease in order to maintain electroneutrality, thus raising the pH. A reduction in water is therefore also referred to as *hypovolemic alkalosis*. Typical causes of increases in sodium concentration due to hypovolemia are diabetes insipidus, vomiting, diarrhea and osmotic diuresis. Conversely, an increase in pure water, which leads to dilution and therefore to a lower Na⁺ concentration, induces, according to the law of electroneutrality, an increase in H⁺. This is why an increase in water is also called *hypervolemic acidosis*. Typical causes are hyperadrenocorticism, administration of hypertonic saline fluid or sodium bicarbonate fluid, and common salt poisoning.

Chapter 2 ◆ Acid–Base Disorders

Chloride, in the body, is in balance with bicarbonate, so that if chloride is reduced bicarbonate is retained and vice versa. The relation between the two ions, however, is not quantitative, because the buffer system is not only made up of bicarbonate, but also of other bases that have negative charges. The amount of chloride also depends on the amount of water available, so its effect must be compensated for by the concentration of sodium (see Tables 2.4 and 2.5). Reductions in chloride levels may be due to vomiting, administration of fluids containing more sodium than chloride (0.9% NaCl solution or sodium bicarbonate), administration of furosemide, hyperadrenocorticism and hyperaldosteronism (which induce sodium retention). Albumin, on the other hand, behaves like a weak acid because it has a negative charge and induces a higher concentration of H^+ ions; its reduction has an alkalizing effect, while its increase has an acidifying effect. In some patients, hypoalbuminemia may occur to compensate for chronic respiratory acidosis; in these cases, the body, which is not able to completely eliminate CO_2, tries to compensate for respiratory acidosis with hypoalbuminemic alkalosis (which reduces the concentration of albumin). Lactate is derived from lactic acid, and for 1 mole of lactic acid 1 mole of H^+ is produced, so an increase in lactate should be interpreted as a sign of increase in an acidic chemical species. Phosphates and sulfates are normally excreted through the kidneys. Their increase is therefore an indicator of impaired renal function; in addition, as they are acidic chemical species, i.e., they have negative charges, their increase causes an increase in H^+. Because they have a negative charge, sulfates promote an acidifying effect, but they are not usually measured in clinical practice. An increase in sulfates is one of the causes of an elevated AG in metabolic acidosis due to renal failure.

Reductions in SID cause acidosis and are the most frequent cause of metabolic acidosis. Typical causes of a reduced SID are diarrhea, duodenal vomiting, excessive water retention (hypervolemic acidosis) caused by congestive heart failure, cavitary effusions, hyperadrenocorticism and the administration of unbalanced electrolyte solutions. Hyperchloremic acidosis can be the consequence of diarrhea (loss of bicarbonate from the intestine with a compensatory increase in chloride), renal failure and, rarely, excessive administration of potassium chloride.

Fluid therapy and SID

When administering fluids, it is important to consider the patient's SID. For example, administration of a large volume of fluid (e.g., liberal fluid management) with a different SID to that of blood can cause an alteration of the patient's SID, and considering that a reduction in the SID is the main factor responsible for changes in pH, its incorrect evaluation can be the cause of a patient's acid–base disturbances. The blood SID, under normal conditions, is about 24. For this reason, when large volumes of fluids are to be administered, it is preferable to choose fluids with an appropriate

Chapter 2 ◆ Acid–Base Disorders

SID instead of considering only the concentration of chloride and other elements. When fluids are administered in large volumes or for a long period, it is advisable to use balanced solutions with a SID of about 24, which are usually obtained by adding molecules with a negative charge and buffer capacity to sodium; instead of chloride alone (such as 0.9% NaCl), acetate, lactate, malate, or gluconate are usually used as anions, so that, instead of reducing the SID, these can behave as *buffers* (increasing the SID). In fact, it should be remembered that some of these ions, in vivo, have a different behavior: for example, solutions containing lactate should theoretically be acidifying because lactate is negatively charged, but because lactate is mainly transformed into a buffer by the liver, in vivo it behaves as an alkalizing solution rather than as an acidifying solution. Bicarbonate is not typically used as it requires glass bottles and can produce vasodilation and calcium carbonate if calcium is present in the solution. Sodium bicarbonate is incompatible with some drugs, such as epinephrine, amoxicillin and clavulanic acid, dobutamine, ketamine, morphine, midazolam, norepinephrine tartrate, ondasentron, and chloride verapamil.

Solutions that have an SID of about 24 should theoretically be neutral from the acid–base point of view, but in reality, altering A_{tot}, they should have a greater SID, or rather a SID comparable to that of the patient, while a solution with a SID of 40–50 should preferably be used when attempting to correct a metabolic acidosis. Colloidal solutions can also affect the SID because they contain A_{tot} in different concentrations, such as gelatin and albumin, while hydroxyethyl starches depend on the solution in which they are dissolved (see Table 2.1 and Table 3.8 in Chapter 3). In general, for maintenance fluid therapy and especially when dealing with hyperchloremic acidosis, it is recommended to use solutions with a high SID or one that is at least greater than that of the patient's plasma, even in the postoperative period, which is generally characterized by metabolic acidosis. When there is no acid–base alteration and the SID is normal, it is preferable to use solutions with an SID similar to that of the patient's plasma.

Clinical case, example

A clinical case interpreted with the traditional and nontraditional approach is described below.

The patient is a male German Shepherd of 5 months of age suffering from sepsis (suspected parvovirosis in its gastrointestinal form), with the following laboratory values:
- pH: 6.8;
- $PaCO_2$: 22 mmHg;
- HCO_3^-: 3.4 mEq/L;
- PaO_2: 98 mmHg;
- lactate: 7.0 mmol/L;

Chapter 2 ◆ Acid–Base Disorders

- Na^+: 150 mEq/L;
- K^+: 3.4 mEq/L;
- Cl^-: 98 mEq/L;
- phosphates: 3.0 mEq/L;
- AG: 28;
- BE: –34.52;
- albumin: 0.9 g/dL;
- hemoglobin: 14.2 g/dL;
- FiO_2: 0.4.

According to the traditional approach, the patient has a mixed disorder, because he has a severe metabolic acidosis: the pH is decreased, with a reduction in HCO_3^- and a severe reduction in BE; in addition, respiratory alkalosis is present. The expected respiratory compensation should bring CO_2 to about 36.6 mmHg, but its value is 22 mmHg.

This means the patient is suffering from hyperventilation and mixed acid–base disorders, since the body never compensates in excess; another morbid process (e.g., pain, anemia) causing hyperventilation and a reduction in CO_2 must therefore be present. The increased AG is likely the consequence of the presence of lactate in the blood as a result of hypovolemic shock.

According to the nontraditional approach, the patient has severe metabolic acidosis (due to a likely increase in lactates) and hypoproteinemic and hyperchloremic alkalosis. In addition, there is an excess of UAs (–26,5). The SID, which should normally be about 29.1 mEq/L, is about 52.6 mEq/L in the patient. The A_{tot}, which should be about 17.4 mEq/L, are about 5 mEq/L. It is therefore a case of severe metabolic acidosis, confirmed by the high concentration of UAs. A metabolic alkalosis is also present due to hypoalbuminemia and hypochloremia; the patient's acidosis is therefore more severe than the pH seems to indicate, because it is "masked" by hypoalbuminemia and hypochloremia. This patient has an H^+ concentration of about 158 nmol/L (under normal conditions, it should be about 34 nmol/L). Hypoalbuminemia reduce the H^+ concentration by about 42 nmol/L, while respiratory alkalosis compensates for acidosis to an extent of about 40 nmol/L.

Table 2.6 Calculation of the effect of strong ions on the base excess

Na^+	0.25 × (150 – 145)	1.25
Cl^-	110 – (98 × 145/150)	10.78
Albumin	3.7 × (3.1 – 0.9)	8.14
Phosphates	0.58 × (5.0 – 3.0)	1.16
Lactate	–1 × [7]	–7
Effect of unmeasured anions (UAs)	UAs = –34.52 – (1.25 + 10.78 + 8.14 + 1.16 + [–7]) UAs = –20.19	

Chapter 2 ◆ Acid–Base Disorders

As shown in this case, when dealing with metabolic acidosis it is necessary to pay attention to the concentrations of albumin, A_{tot} and chloride (the latter because it could aggravate metabolic acidosis).

By calculating each component and subtracting it from the BE, the values listed in Table 2.6 are obtained for each component.

From the calculation of the strong ions reported in Table 2.6, the severe acidosis is evident, given the presence of a considerable amount of UAs, and of an alkalosis from hypoalbuminemia and hypochloremia, although there is also an alkalosis from SID that compensates for it.

Strong ion gap (SIG)

The SIG is another quantitative approach to determining the presence of UAs in dogs and cats. According to this theory, the net sum of strong ions (sodium, potassium, calcium, magnesium, from which chloride and lactate are subtracted) must be balanced by the activity of anions (albumin, total proteins and phosphorus). The simplified SIG is measured using the following formulas:

$$SIG = [alb] \times 4.9 - AG \text{ (dog)} \qquad (Equation\ 14)$$

$$SIG = [alb] \times 7.4 - AG \text{ (cat)} \qquad (Equation\ 15)$$

[alb], measured albumin concentration; $AG = (Na^+ + K^+) - (Cl^- + HCO_3^-)$.
In the presence of hyperphosphatemia, the AG must be corrected: correct $AG = AG + (2.52 - 0.58 \times [phosphate])$

Values below –5 or –6 suggest the presence of UAs; values above +5 or +6 suggest the presence of UCs (unmeasured cations), an event that occurs rarely. The cause for a reduction in the SIG below the normal range should be promptly investigated and treated.

Correction of acid–base disorders

The possible acid–base disorders are as follows:
- metabolic acidosis;
- metabolic alkalosis;
- respiratory acidosis;
- respiratory alkalosis;
- mixed, respiratory and metabolic disorders:

Chapter 2 ◆ Acid–Base Disorders

- respiratory acidosis and metabolic alkalosis;
- respiratory and metabolic acidosis;
- respiratory alkalosis and metabolic acidosis;
- respiratory and metabolic alkalosis;
- metabolic acidosis and metabolic alkalosis;
- respiratory acidosis and respiratory alkalosis;
- metabolic acidosis with normal or increased AG;
- metabolic acidosis with elevated AG;
- metabolic acidosis with normal AG;
- triple disorders.

Metabolic acidosis

Metabolic acidosis consists in a decreased pH (<7,4) and can be caused by a decrease in bicarbonate or an increase in hydrogen ions; it is characterized by a secondary compensatory respiratory alkalosis (decreased $PaCO_2$). The most common causes of metabolic acidosis are summarized in Table 2.3.

Treatment of metabolic acidosis

The treatment of metabolic acidosis should primarily aim to treat the morbid process that caused the acid–base disorders (see Table 2.3). To this end, the primary disorder must be identified, so we must ensure that there is no alteration caused or modified by strong ions that control the SID, A_{tot}, phosphates and sulfates. The etiology of metabolic acidosis is variable and a specific therapy will be needed in each case, but all types of metabolic acidosis will have to be treated with balanced isotonic solutions containing bicarbonate precursors (e.g., lactate or acetate). The choice of the type of solution will depend on the patient's electrolytes and blood pH. Generally, treating the cause of acidosis, restoring the lost volume, and continuing with maintenance fluid therapy using isotonic crystalloids that contain bicarbonate precursors (e.g., electrolyte replenishment solution with sodium gluconate or acetated Ringer's solution) will correct metabolic acidosis. After restoring the lost volume and starting maintenance fluid therapy, it is advised to repeat the ABG after at least 30 minutes. In some cases of severe metabolic acidosis, such as those caused by chronic kidney failure, an alkalizing treatment with sodium bicarbonate will be necessary.

Sodium bicarbonate therapy

An alkalizing treatment with sodium bicarbonate should be considered in patients with a pH below 7.2, a BE below –10 mEq/L and bicarbonate levels below 14 mEq/L. When the pH reaches values below 7.0, the acid–base disorder can impair vital functions and must be treated urgently and aggressively, not with sodium bicarbonate but

Chapter 2 ♦ Acid–Base Disorders

with alkalizing solutions, given that bicarbonate infusion can be fatal it is performed too quickly (<20 min).

The alkalizing effect of $NaHCO_3^-$ is also obtained thanks to the large amount of sodium present in the solution: as it is a strong cation, it induces a reduction in H^+. An 8.4% solution contains 1000 mEq/L of $NaHCO_3^-$ and thus has a SID of 1000. The dose of bicarbonate to be administered is calculated using the following equation:

$$0.3 \times kg \times (\text{ideal } HCO_3^- - \text{patient } HCO_3^-) = HCO_3^- \text{ to be administered}$$

(Equation 16)

Approximately 1/4 or 1/2 of the calculated dose should be administered at a rate greater than that necessary to be redistributed from the intravascular compartment to the interstitial compartment, i.e., in about 20–30 minutes. Faster administration can cause cardiovascular collapse and death of the patient. In the absence of an ABG, the empirical dose that is sometimes used is 1–5 mEq/kg, and corresponds to the amount needed to correct an approximate deficit of 5–15 mEq/L. This method is dangerous as not knowing the required amount of sodium bicarbonate that should be administered can be the cause of iatrogenic alkalosis.

Before administering sodium bicarbonate, it is necessary to check the patient's ability to ventilate, as it is important that the CO_2 produced as a result of this treatment can be eliminated through ventilation; CO_2 is then rapidly excreted, which generates an excess of intracellular H^+ (paradoxical acidosis), responsible for the depression of the CNS and myocardial function. Patients with normal ventilation only require a few ventilatory cycles to eliminate excess CO_2.

Rapid administration of bicarbonate or excessive alkalinization can cause nausea, vomiting, hypotension, collapse, and death. The cause of such effects lies in the rapid alteration of the H^+ concentration, with a reduction in potassium and calcium ion levels. The administration of sodium bicarbonate also causes hypernatremia, especially when repeated doses are administered; it is therefore necessary to perform another ABG at least 30 minutes after its administration.

Sodium bicarbonate solution is hypertonic (2000 mOsm/kg) and it can cause vascular irritation and pain when infused peripherally. To reduce its osmolality, it is possible to dilute one part of sodium bicarbonate in 6.5 parts of 5% dextrose solution, which will reduce natremia (154 mEq/L) and make the solution iso-osmolar (308 mOsm/L).

Metabolic alkalosis

Metabolic alkalosis consists of an increase in pH (>7.45) and bicarbonate (>24 mEq/L) associated with a reduction in H^+. It is characterized by a compensatory increase in

Chapter 2 ♦ Acid–Base Disorders

CO_2. Metabolic alkalosis is less frequent than metabolic acidosis and it is often associated with hypokalemia and hypovolemia. The most common cause of alkalosis is the loss of hydrogen ions due to vomiting, more rarely to urine excretion or the administration of diuretics; it can also develop after hypercapnia.

After diagnosing alkalosis, it is necessary to ensure that no alteration has been caused or modified by strong ions by checking sodium, chloride, protein (especially albumin), phosphate and sulfate levels. In particular, chloremia must be verified, because its reduction is the cause of alkalosis; it is frequently produced by the loss of gastroenteric fluids (e.g., following vomiting and diarrhea), which contain large quantities of chloride. Iatrogenic alkalosis rarely occurs due to administration of alkalis as the body can eliminate them. When this phenomenon occurs, kidney function must be controlled.

Alkalosis is frequently associated with potassium losses (e.g., following vomiting). In this case, intracellular potassium moves out of cells to compensate for the losses and electroneutrality is maintained by the movement of sodium and hydrogen ions into cells, which produces extracellular alkalosis and intracellular acidosis. Compensatory hypochloremia (to achieve electroneutrality) resulting from an increase in extracellular negative charges aggravates alkalosis, thus reducing the possibility of anion reabsorption in the renal proximal tubules. Sodium and potassium are reabsorbed into cells, which causes hypokalemia. Bicarbonate binds to the hydrogen ions moving out of the cell to form carbonic acid; this generates CO_2, which must be eliminated through ventilation. Large losses of extravascular volume (e.g., due to incoercible vomiting or duodenal diarrhea) favor sodium and bicarbonate ion reabsorption by the renal proximal tubules, the movement of potassium into the lumen of the tubules (which is then excreted with urine), and metabolic alkalosis.

During therapy with furosemide, alkalosis may occur due to extracellular fluid contraction, as the loss of chloride ions is compensated for by an increase in bicarbonate. Under normal conditions this effect is compensated for by the activity of the normal cell membrane and bones, but in case of renal failure this phenomenon is more severe.

Metabolic alkaloses can be classified into two types: with severe extracellular fluid (ECF) depletion and with normal ECF. The former alkaloses respond to chloride therapy (administration of NaCl 0.9%), while the latter do not and are less frequent and caused by hyperaldosteronism or hyperadrenocorticism.

The most common causes of metabolic alkalosis are the following:
- gastric diseases;
- vomiting;
- aspiration of gastric contents;
- hypochloremia (e.g., from diarrhea);
- hypokalemia;

Chapter 2 ◆ Acid–Base Disorders

- administration of mineralocorticoids;
- administration of furosemide or thiazide diuretics;
- hypomineralcorticism;
- metabolism of citrate and ketone bodies;
- administration of carbenicillin or penicillin derivatives;
- administration of antacids;
- contraction alkalosis;
- alkalizing therapy;
- compensation of respiratory acidosis.

Treatment of metabolic alkalosis

The treatment of metabolic alkalosis depends on the type of alkalosis (chloride-responsive or non-chloride-responsive). With the first type it is necessary to administer acidifying crystalloid solutions such as 0.9% NaCl; with the second type (hyperaldosteronism or hyperadrenocorticism), the morbid process must be treated. In patients with imbalances that respond to chloride therapy, volemia should be restored with 0.9% NaCl solution; this ensures losses (dehydration) are replenished and hypokalemia is treated. After this initial phase of fluid therapy, an ABG should be performed to check the effectiveness of the treatment. When the arterial pH is between 7.4 and 7.65, it is sufficient to treat the morbid process that caused the disorder (e.g., by controlling vomiting) and initiate fluid therapy with isotonic saline solution. A pH greater than 7.65 requires a more aggressive treatment with acidifying fluid therapy (0.9% NaCl with added KCl) and close monitoring of the patient. If the pH is above 7.8, immediate therapy is required as this value is incompatible with life. Fluid therapy with 0.9% NaCl solution should always be supplemented with potassium chloride (see Chapter 3) in order to correct hypokalemia.

Respiratory acidosis

Respiratory acidosis is the consequence of insufficient ventilation, responsible for an increase in CO_2. It is characterized by a reduction in pH and a compensatory increase in blood bicarbonate concentration. In chronic forms, there may be a reduction in total protein or albumin, or both. This disturbance is caused by an inability of the body to eliminate CO_2 due to airway stenosis (e.g., asthma, pleural effusion) or impaired ventilatory function (e.g., CNS diseases). In the body, the CO_2 produced can be eliminated through ventilation or combine with the hemoglobin in red blood cells to form carbaminohemoglobin.

The causes of respiratory acidosis are as follows:
- alterations of CNS activity: head trauma, general anesthesia, opioids, neoplasms;

- diseases of the peripheral nervous system: tetanus, botulism, organophosphates, hypokalemia, tick paralysis, polyradicoloneuritis, polymyositis, phrenic nerve dysfunction, myasthenia gravis;
- injuries of the chest wall: trauma, rib fractures, pleural effusions;
- lung diseases: pneumonia, asthma, pulmonary thromboembolism, severe pulmonary edema, smoke inhalation;
- airway obstructions: diseases of the pleural space, diaphragmatic hernia, pneumothorax, pleural effusions, laryngospasm, tracheal collapse, laryngeal paralysis, brachycephalic syndrome, asthma;
- ineffective mechanical ventilation;
- increased CO_2 production: heatstroke, malignant hyperthermia, cardiopulmonary arrest.

Respiratory acidosis can be acute (e.g., pneumothorax) or chronic (e.g., feline asthma). Chronic acidosis can be compensated for by renal retention of bicarbonate ions, while acute acidosis cannot benefit from this compensatory mechanism because the kidneys need several hours to initiate bicarbonate ion retention (which culminates within 2–5 days). Chronic acidosis can be compensated for by a decrease in albumin, which, because of its negative charge, can reduce the H^+ concentration.

During respiratory acidosis, in addition to compensation with retention of bicarbonate ions, the body buffers excess hydrogen ions with basic phosphate to form phosphoric acid, and with blood proteins.

Excess hydrogen ions enter the cells by exchanging with potassium, thus causing hypokalemia. Increased CO_2 is often associated with hypoxia, which is why some severe cases of respiratory acidosis, if not treated with oxygen therapy, can be fatal. In these patients, oxygen therapy is provided (when the partial pressure of oxygen is ≤80 mmHg or oxygenated hemoglobin falls below 95%), although the administration of oxygen cannot reduce CO_2 because it does not improve ventilation if it is impaired; in fact, it improves it only in case of hypoxia.

When hypercapnia is not corrected, patients show respiratory distress, reduced cardiac output and blood pressure, depression of the CNS and loss of consciousness.

Treatment of respiratory acidosis

Treatment begins with the diagnosis of acute hypercapnia, as this should be treated as early as possible (e.g., with chest drainage or positive pressure ventilation). In all cases it is advisable to also provide oxygen therapy, from the moment the patient is admitted until the treatment is initiated to reduce cerebral hypoxia. In acute and severe forms (e.g., laryngeal paralysis, brachycephalic syndrome, severe tracheal collapse), it is necessary to induce anesthesia and emergency orotracheal intubation or tracheostomy in order to perform positive pressure ventilation; in chronic forms, appropriate diagnostic investigations must be performed to identify the morbid process and take the most appropriate therapeutic measures. Chronic respiratory acidosis leads to compensatory metabolic alkalosis, but this latter can also be of iatrogenic origin as a result of the administration of diuretics and corticosteroids.

In hypercapnic patients, excessive oxygen administration can suppress the hypoxic reflex, which is the natural ventilatory stimulus, so when adequate oxygenation is achieved (PaO_2 >80 mmHg or oxygenated hemoglobin >95%) aggressive ventilation should be discontinued.

Fluid therapy should consist of balanced isotonic solutions containing bicarbonate precursors; when it is associated with correction of the main problem, it is usually sufficient to correct acidosis. Bicarbonate administration is not recommended as it can increase the SID and ultimately reduce the pH, as well as reduce the ventilatory stimulus and aggravate hypoxia with an increase in CO_2, which will in turn aggravate acidosis because the patient is not able to eliminate the increased fraction of CO_2 resulting from bicarbonate administration.

Respiratory alkalosis

Respiratory alkalosis involves decreased CO_2 and is characterized by an increase in pH and a compensatory reduction in bicarbonate. It is the result of an increase in ventilation that exceeds the production of CO_2. The causes of hyperventilation are hypoxemia (e.g., right-to-left shunts, congestive heart failure), tissue hypoxia without hypoxemia (e.g., anemia, hypotension, carboxyhemoglobin), shock, SIRS (systemic inflammatory response syndrome), acute lung diseases (e.g., pneumonia, thromboembolism, pulmonary edema, ARDS), and stimulation of receptors located in the CNS (e.g., pain, trauma, infections, liver disease, resolution of metabolic acidosis, pregnancy, salicylate poisoning and heatstroke).

Treatment of respiratory alkalosis

The treatment of respiratory alkalosis requires rapid diagnosis and treatment of its cause. Generally, treatment of hypoxia (oxygen therapy) is sufficient to correct hyperventilation. In cases refractory to oxygen therapy, i.e., when the PaO_2 is <60 mmHg or hemoglobin saturation remains ≤90%, positive pressure ventilation is required. Respiratory alkalosis can also result from pain: in these cases, the administration of analgesic drugs corrects the acid–base imbalance.

Mixed disorders

Mixed acid–base disorders occur when two or more primary disorders (e.g., triple disorders) develop at the same time. A typical example is a patient with chronic renal failure who may have a pH close to normal due to a metabolic alkalosis from vomiting (e.g., due to gastric mucosal erosion) and a simultaneous acidosis due to loss of bicarbonate ions resulting from renal failure.

Chapter 2 ◆ Acid–Base Disorders

Mixed disorders should always be suspected when the pH is normal or close to normal while the metabolic (bicarbonate) and respiratory (carbon dioxide) components have opposite directions and values beyond normal compensation. The definitive diagnosis is made by identifying the different acid–base disturbances. In summary, the suggestive alterations of a mixed disorder are:
- a normal pH with changes in $PaCO_2$ and HCO_3^- in the opposite direction;
- a change in pH in the opposite direction from the primary disorder;
- alterations of the metabolic and respiratory components beyond the expected compensation;
- changes in metabolic and respiratory components in the same direction.

Treatment of mixed disorders

The treatment of mixed disorders should be aimed at treating the primary disorder. The first step is therefore to diagnose and correct the main problem, before repeating the ABG. If secondary disorders have not normalized, they must be corrected (e.g., by fluid therapy and correction of electrolyte or respiratory disorders). For example, if, in a patient with pneumothorax, diagnosed with a respiratory alkalosis and a circulatory failure due to a reduction in cardiac output resulting from the increase in intrathoracic pressure, a perfusion deficiency is still observed after the air has been removed with a thoracic drainage, then it is advisable to administer resuscitation fluids. If these fluids had been administered before drainage, they could have been ineffective or have further impaired ventilation due to pulmonary overload. In summary, the most severe disease process should be treated first, as it can compromise the patient's vital functions, and only then should the other disturbances be corrected if they are still present. Generally, correction of the main disorder and administration of balanced isotonic solutions (chosen based on the results of the assessment of the acid–base and electrolyte status) are sufficient to correct mixed disorders.

Suggested readings

[1] Rose BD. Introduction to simple and mixed acid base disorder. In Rose BD, Post TW (eds.). *Clinical physiology of acid-base and electrolyte disorders*, 5th ed. New York: McGraw Hill; 2001. pp. 535–550.

[2] Martin L. *All you really need to know to interpret arterial blood gases*. Philadelphia: Lippincott Williams & Wilkins; 1999.

[3] DiBartola SP. *Fluid, electrolyte, and acid-base disorders in small animal practice*, 4th ed. St. Louis: Elsevier Saunders; 2011.

[4] Hahn RG. *Clinical fluid therapy in the perioperative setting*. Cambridge: Cambridge University Press; 2016.

Clinical Case

The cat who couldn't urinate

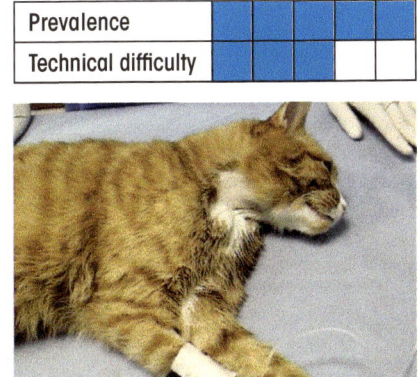

Prevalence	■	■	■	■
Technical difficulty	■	■		

Signalment	
Name	Red
Species	feline
Breed	European shorthair
Sex	male
Weight	3.8 kg
Age	3 years

Clinical history

The patient is presented to the clinic due to stranguria; he has not been eating or drinking for 2 days and is continuously licking his foreskin, where some blood loss can be observed. His last stool was normal. He is restless and does not want to be held by his owner or anyone who approaches.

At triage, the following vital parameters are assessed:
- heart rate: 180 bpm;
- respiratory rate: 52 bpm;
- pulse: normal;
- rectal temperature: 39.3 °C;
- mucous membranes: pink, CRT <1.5 seconds;
- blood pressure: 180/120 mmHg, MAP: 140 mmHg;
- dehydration: absent;
- pain on abdominal palpation and presence of a distended bladder.

Chapter 2 ◆ Acid–Base Disorders

Laboratory tests

A blood gas analysis is performed as part of the laboratory tests, as a urethral obstruction is suspected with possible electrolyte complications, in particular a risk of hyperkalemia. In these cases, it is important to know the acid–base and electrolyte status, because potential hyperkalemia could compromise vital functions. A complete blood count is also performed to assess hematological parameters and the likelihood of an infection. A biochemical profile is used to evaluate the possible presence of kidney or other organ dysfunction and to check whether, using the nontraditional approach to acid–base disorders, other metabolic components are involved.

Venous blood gas analysis

Given that there is no disease of the respiratory system, venous sampling is performed, since venous blood gas analysis is a reliable way of measuring pH, bicarbonate, carbon dioxide and electrolytes.
- pH: 7.10;
- $pvCO_2$: 39;
- HCO_3^-: 12;
- BE: –17;
- Na^+: 150 mmol/L;
- Cl^-: 121 mmol/L;
- K^+: 7.3 mmol/L;
- lactate: 1.4 mmol/L;
- AG: 26.8;
- FiO2: 0.21.

Biochemical profile

BUN >300 mg/dL, creatinine 9.3 mg/dL, ALT 32 U/L, AST 12 U/L, total protein 4.2 g/dL, albumin 1.0 g/dL, total bilirubin 0.01 mg/dL, GGT 2 U/L, glucose 153 mg/100 mL, phosphorus 9.4 mg/dL.

Clinical Case

Complete blood count

RBC 5.9 × 10^{12}/L, WBC 8.5 × 10^9/L, Hct 34%, Hb 11.0 g/dL, PLT 245 × 10^9/L, neutrophils 10 × 10^3/μL.

Interpretation of laboratory tests

The blood gas analysis shows a metabolic acidosis and a compensatory respiratory alkalosis; CO_2 reflects the expected value of compensation: it had to be reduced by about 10 units. Bicarbonate is very low and corresponds to the primary disturbance, as it goes in the same direction as pH. The cause probably lies in postrenal acute kidney injury due to urinary tract obstruction.

According to the nontraditional approach, a severe acidosis and mild SID alkalosis (-6 nmol/L) are present. There is also an A_{tot} alkalosis that contributes in about –22 nmol/L acidity, given that the severe acidosis is caused by unmeasured anions. Severe hyperkalemia is present and could lead to fatal arrythmias. The biochemical profile reveals a very severely increased BUN and serum creatinine probably of postrenal origin. The complete blood count shows a mild anemia, which is probably due to chronic hematuria.

Osmolarity is calculated as follows:

$$Osm = 2 \times [Na^+] + glucose\ (mg/dL)/18 + BUN\ (mg/dL)/2.8$$

$$Osm = (2 \times 150) + (153/18) + (300/2.8)$$

$$Osm = 416\ mOsm/L$$

Osmolarity is higher than normal due to the slight increase in natremia, but especially as a result of severe azotemia. Control of osmolality will be achieved, more than with fluid therapy, by treating the urethral obstruction, which will reduce azotemia and therefore the osmotic pressure of blood.

Chapter 2 ◆ Acid–Base Disorders

Diagnostic tests

An X-ray of the abdomen is taken and reveals a distended urinary bladder and numerous bladder stones.

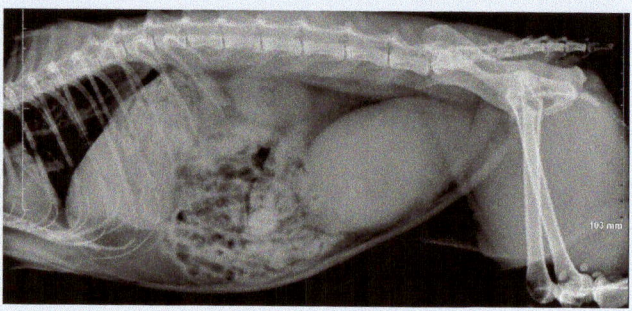

Daily fluid therapy

Maintenance fluid therapy with a high SID should be provided to try to correct the severe metabolic acidosis. Since the patient is not dehydrated and is not suffering from any other losses, administration of the maintenance fluid volume only is sufficient.

Maintenance fluid therapy: 2 mL/kg/hour IV, which corresponds to 8 mL/hour. The solution chosen for the patient is a balanced polyelectrolyte solution with sodium gluconate, as it contains 50 bicarbonate precursors (SID equal to 50). If the previous solution is not available, it is also possible to administer lactated or acetated Ringer's solution; although these solutions contain potassium, this does not affect the outcome of the treatment of the morbid process, because the most critical element is to resolve the urethral obstruction as quickly as possible. Before treating the urethral obstruction, an electrocardiogram is performed that does not show any rhythm alterations, only a sinus tachycardia and a slight elevation of the T wave, with the first abnormality probably being due to pain and agitation caused by handling.

Clinical Case

Treatment of urethral obstruction

To unblock the urethra, the patient is put under general anesthesia by gas after induction by intramuscular administration of 10 mg/kg ketamine and 0.4 mg/kg midazolam in the same syringe, followed by oxygen therapy and mask induction with 2.5% isoflurane. Once the induction is complete, the patient is intubated and the urethra is unblocked.

The urethra is easily unblocked by placing a bladder catheter. A high amount of blood is present in the urine drained by the catheter, thus prompting the decision to leave the catheter until this amount is reduced; if this is not done, the presence of a considerable amount of blood could cause a new urethral obstruction. The bladder catheter is then removed on day 2.

In this case, only a slight elevation of the T wave was observed on the electrocardiogram, but if more severe abnormalities had been detected, 2 mL of 10% calcium gluconate could have been administered to the patient by slow intravenous infusion. The following day the patient starts eating and drinking again spontaneously, so the blood gas analysis and biochemical profile are repeated with the following results:

- pH: 7.45;
- $pvCO_2$: 42;
- HCO_3^-: 22;
- BE: 4.2;
- Na^+: 143 mmol/L;
- Cl^-: 121 mmol/L;
- K^+: 3.5 mmol/L;
- lactate: 0.4 mmol/L;
- AG: 3.5;
- FiO_2: 0.21.

The biochemical profile shows the following results: BUN 54 mg/dL, creatinine 3.8 mg/dL, ALT 45 U/L, AST 23 U/L, total proteins 3.8 g/dL, albumin 1.2 g/dL, total bilirubin 0.02 mg/dL, GGT 2 U/L, blood glucose 97 mg/100 mL, phosphate 6.5 mg/dL.

The patient is discharged on day 3 with a diet to dissolve stones and supplements for restoring the integrity of the bladder mucosa.

Fluids: when and how to administer them

Fabio Viganò

Introduction

The administration of fluids, like that of any other drug, has its indications and contraindications; however, unlike with other drugs, fluid therapy requires an evaluation of the water and electrolyte balance and of the hemodynamic effects that it can produce. When administering fluid therapy, the following priorities must be followed:
- identifying the patient's needs;
- establishing the objectives to be achieved;
- performing hemodynamic monitoring;
- performing electrolytic and acid–base monitoring.

Fluid therapy is indicated to maintain hydration, restore an effective circulating volume (resuscitative fluid therapy), and achieve correct rehydration.

Daily intravenous fluid therapy

Under normal conditions, the patient's water requirements are satisfied by the ingestion of water and food. However, when, due to some pathological processes, the patient cannot take anything by mouth, it is necessary to replace the physiological intake of water and electrolytes by the administration of fluids to maintain the hydration status and replace ongoing losses. Normally, the body loses water through the feces and urine. These losses are defined as sensitive and measurable. Other losses, which occur through breathing and sweating, are defined as insensitive and are not easily measurable; they typically do not cause significant electrolyte losses. Like sensitive losses, insensitive losses can become clinically relevant and aggravate dehydration, for example, when the respiratory rate increases due to hyperthermia or in case of pulmonary hypertension. Since sweating in dogs and cats is negligible, it cannot cause water and electrolyte imbalances as is the case, for example, in horses.

Chapter 3 ◆ Fluids: when and how to administer them

Daily water requirements

The NRC (National Research Council of the United States) has established, based on a review of the literature [1], that the water requirements of dogs, expressed in mL, correspond to kcal (1 kcal = 1 mL), using a range of values between 94 and 183 multiplied by the metabolic weight, as shown in the following equation:

$$94 / 183 \times kg^{0.75} \qquad (Equation\ 1)$$

The NRC has also established water requirements for cats, which correspond to about 0.6–0.7 mL per kcal, calculated based on energy requirements ranging from 31 to 100 kcal/kg for a total of about 22–70 mL/kg/day. The needs calculated by the NRC are based on healthy patients, so a sick animal that is unable to move is likely to have reduced water requirements. In addition, it should be remembered that the oxidation of 100 g of fat generates about 100 mL of water, while that of 100 g of carbohydrates generates 60 mL of water, and that of 100 g of protein generates 40 mL of water. In a recent study in veterinary medicine [2], the authors recommended using the following equation to calculate daily water requirements:

$$97 \times kg^{0.655} \qquad (Equation\ 2)$$

Another method to determine daily water requirements in dogs and cats is to apply the equation used to calculate calorie requirements, assuming that the caloric and water needs in mL are equivalent:

$$30 \times kg + 70 \qquad (Equation\ 3)$$

In patients weighing less than 2 kg, the equation that considers the metabolic weight can be used:

$$70 \times kg^{0.75} \qquad (Equation\ 4)$$

Another method for a very quick calculation of water needs is to estimate them based on kg of body weight and administer fluids at a rate of 1.2–2.0 mL/kg/hour intravenously. The lower values should be used in large or giant dogs, while the higher values should be used in small or dehydrated patients. This method, which is very quick and simple, can be used at first, but it is always recommended, as with the other methods, to constantly monitor the patient's clinical, hemodynamic, and laboratory parameters to evaluate the effectiveness or toxicity of the volume of fluids administered.

Chapter 3 ◆ Fluids: when and how to administer them

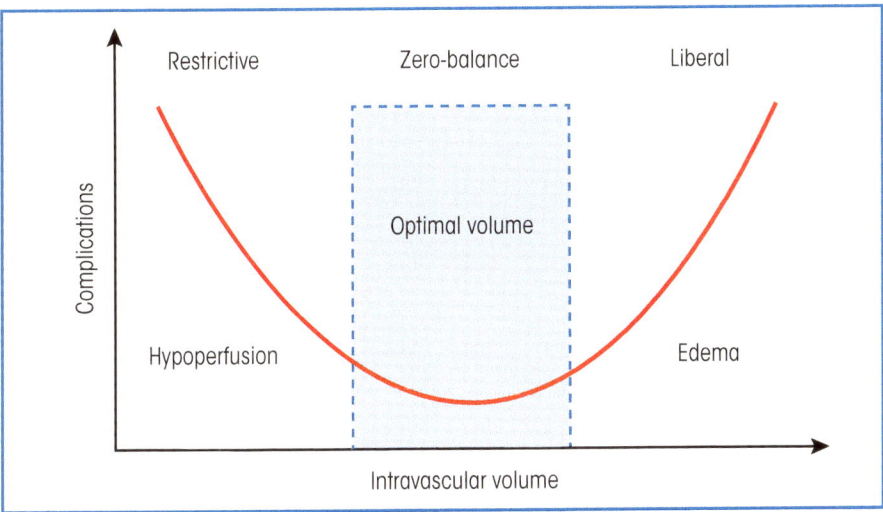

Figure 3.1 Fluid volume and complications.

Therefore, daily fluid therapy should avoid the risks and complications resulting from hypovolemia, such as hypoperfusion, organ dysfunction, and an unfavorable outcome of the ongoing pathological process; on the other hand, an excess of fluids can cause edema, in addition to organ dysfunction and unfavorable outcome (Figure 3.1).

Daily fluid therapy can be provided using balanced solutions, which have a similar composition and osmolarity to those of plasma, or hypotonic solutions, which have a lower electrolyte content than balanced solutions in order to reduce the likelihood of causing water retention and electrolyte imbalances (Table 3.1). Electrolyte and water requirements in dogs and cats have been established by the NRC [1] and are summarized in Tables 3.2 and 3.3. For the calculation of daily maintenance water requirements, see Box 3.1.

Hypotonic solutions

For maintenance fluid therapy, in addition to establishing the amount of fluids that should be administered daily (see above), it is necessary to determine the tonicity the solution should have and, therefore, how much sodium it should contain; its appropriate SID (strong ion difference), i.e., how many bicarbonate precursors and how many electrolytes such as potassium and chloride it should contain; and whether glucose or other electrolytes should be added.

Chapter 3 ◆ Fluids: when and how to administer them

Table 3.1 Composition of crystalloids in 500 mL

Solution	pH	On	Cl⁻	K⁺	Ca²⁺	Mg⁺	Osmolarity (mOsm/L)	Kcal/L	Buffer (mOsm/L)	SID
Plasma	7.4	145	103	5	0	3	295	0	22	24
0.9% Saline solution	5.0	154	154	0	0	0	308	0	0	0
Plasma-Lyte	5.5–7.0	140	98	5	0	3	0	0	Gluconate 23, Acetate 27	50
Ringer's acetate	6.4	132	109.5	4	3	0	276	0	Acetate 29.5	29.5
Ringer's lactate	6.5	131,5	111.5	5	3,5	0	279	0	Lactate 29	29
Normosol M	4.0–6.5	40	40	13	0	3	363	0	Acetate 16	16
Rehydrating electrolytic III*	5.5	140	103	10	5	3	306	0	Acetate 47	47
Glucion 5%	4.0–5.2	27	27.5	13	0	2.6	443	170	Lactate 12.5	12.5
GNaK	4.5	25.5	45	20	0	0	460	170	0	0
Hypotonax	5.3	12.5	11	10	0	1.5	372	170	12.5	12.5
5% Glucose	4.0	0	0	0	0	0	252	170	0	0
20% Glucose	4.0	0	0	0	0	0	1112	800	0	0
50% Glucose	4.2	0	0	0	0	0	2780	1700	0	0
18% Mannitol	4.5–7.0	0	0	0	0	0	988	0	0	0
3% NaCl	5.0	513	513	0	0	0	1026	0	0	0
7.5% NaCl	5.0	1280	1280	0	0	0	2400	0	0	0

* Elettrolitico reidratante III

Chapter 3 ◆ Fluids: when and how to administer them

Table 3.2 Daily electrolyte and water requirements in dogs and cats

Elements and water	Dog mg/kg$^{0.75}$	mEq/kg$^{0.75}$	Cat mg/kg$^{0.67}$	mEq/kg$^{0.67}$
Sodium	9.85	0.43	16	0.7
Potassium	140	3.59	97	2.49
Chloride	40	1.13	23.7	0.67
Calcium	52	2.6	32	1.6
Magnesium	6	0.49	4.9	0.40
Water	97 × kg$^{0.66}$			

Table 3.3 Examples of daily water and electrolyte requirements in dogs and cats

Elements and water	Dog mEq/kg$^{0.75}$	Dog 10 kg, mEq	Cat mEq/kg$^{0.67}$	Cat 4 kg, mEq	Plasma mEq/L
Sodium	0.43	2.4	0.7	1.8	145
Potassium	3.59	20.2	2.49	6.3	5
Chloride	1.13	6.35	0.67	1.7	105
Calcium	2.6	14.62	1.6	4.1	5
Magnesium	0.49	2.76	0.40	1.0	3
Water		443 mL/day		242 mL/day	

Box 3.1 — Calculation examples for daily water maintenance in mL

- Dogs: $94 / 183 \times kg^{0.75}$
- Dogs and cats: $97 \times kg^{0.655}$
- $30 \times kg + 70$
- $70 \times kg^{0.75}$
- 30–48 mL/kg/day

Chapter 3 ◆ Fluids: when and how to administer them

In human medicine, the following guidelines for daily fluid therapy were established in 2015 [3] (NICE guidelines): 25–30 mL/kg/day of water; 1 mmol/kg/day of sodium, potassium, chloride; and 50–100 g/day of glucose (100 mL of a 5% solution contains 5 g of glucose). In veterinary medicine, guidelines for daily fluid therapy have not yet been established. The risk of administering hypotonic fluids is that these can cause hyponatremia: a study conducted in 690 pediatric human patients [4] who were given a 0.45% solution of NaCl showed a three-fold increase in cases of hyponatremia. In a study [5] in 12 healthy fasted human patients who were administered either hypotonic (Na^+ 50 mEq/L, K^+ 26 mEq/L, Cl^- 55 mEq/L, phosphate 6.2 mEq/L, glucose 50 g/L, lactate 25 mEq/L) or isotonic fluids (Na^+ 154 mEq/L, K^+ 40 mEq/L, Cl^- 194 mEq/L, glucose 50 g/L) for 48 hours, a reduction in urine production, lower production of antidiuretic hormone, and expansion of the circulating volume was observed in the group receiving the isotonic solution, while those patients who had been administered an hypotonic solution developed hyperchloremia with no reduction in the blood concentration of sodium or potassium.

The contradictory studies in human and veterinary medicine do not allow a conclusion to be reached or the establishment of definitive guidelines, and it is therefore recommended, when providing daily fluid therapy and especially when large volumes are administered for several days, to check the patient's body weight (to identify any weight gain or loss from water retention or dehydration) twice a day, the electrolyte concentration and pH at least once a day, and the production of urine over 24 hours. Since balanced saline solutions contain an excess of sodium and chloride, but little potassium, a possible maintenance solution could be as follows: Na^+ 34–51 mEq/L + 5% dextrose + K^+ 40 mEq/L + Mg^+ 8 mEq/L.

Hypotonic solutions low in sodium are available on the market, such as Normosol M® Hospira, which contains Na^+ 40 mEq/L, Cl^- 40 mEq/L, K^+ 13 mEq/L, Mg^+ 3 mEq/L, acetate 16 mEq/L (Osm 363 and pH 4.0–6.5). When looking at its composition, it can easily be seen that this solution is also hyponatremic and hyperkalemic compared to the plasma of our patients, so when it is administered at high rates and for long periods it is advisable to closely monitor the electrolytes, pH and patient's weight.

Antidiuretic hormone and fluid therapy

The effects of ADH (antidiuretic hormone) should also be considered in the daily fluid therapy of critically ill patients, given that in the presence of severe stress, hypovolemia or hypotension, ADH promotes water retention by retaining sodium and thus limiting urine production in an attempt to correct hemodynamic deficits. Therefore, the administration of hypotonic fluids in patients in which ADH release is increased can more easily cause hyponatremia due to the increased water retention induced by ADH.

Chapter 3 ◆ Fluids: when and how to administer them

Fluid therapy under general anesthesia

Even in patients under general anesthesia there is an excess of ADH release, which is insensitive to the administration of fluids [6]. In these patients it is therefore advisable to administer isotonic saline solutions at 2–3 mL/kg/hour IV. In the past, much larger volumes of up to 10 mL/kg/hour IV were used, as it was assumed that this infusion rate was necessary to restore water losses due to evaporation from the exposed viscera during abdominal and thoracic surgery. In humans, water losses through perspiration have been estimated and are proportional to those due to exposure of the viscera, as occurs during abdominal surgery: a small incision with no exteriorization of the viscera (e.g., appendectomy) produces a loss of water of about 2.1 mL/kg/hour, while losses through evaporation are about 8.0 mL/kg/hour with an average incision with partial exteriorization of the viscera (e.g., cholecystectomy), and 32.2 mL/kg/hour with an extended incision with exteriorization of all viscera. Such losses are reduced by 50% after 20 minutes; if the viscera are placed in a plastic bag, losses are reduced by 87%.

A recent study called RELIEF conducted in human patients [7,8] has demonstrated the potential benefits of restrictive fluid therapy during abdominal surgery when compared to liberal fluid therapy [9]. In this study, restrictive fluid therapy involved administering 5 mL/kg of fluids at induction and 5 mL/kg/hour during surgery (lasting at least 2 hours). After surgery, 0.8 mL/kg/hour of fluids were administered and fluid administration was discontinued as early as possible. The control group receiving liberal fluid therapy were administered 10 mL/kg of fluids at induction and 8 mL/kg/hour during surgery (lasting at least 2 hours). After surgery, >1.5 mL/kg/hour of fluids were administered over a period of 24 hours or more (Box 3.2).

Daily fluid therapy

Before calculating the daily fluid therapy, it is essential to establish whether a rapid replacement of the circulating volume is necessary or whether the patient only needs

Box 3.2	Fluid volumes under general anesthesia

- Isotonic saline solution: 2–3 mL/kg/hour
- Fluid bolus: 5 mL/kg/5 min (if not due to vasodilation)
- Hemorrhage: isotonic saline solution 3:1 lost blood volume

Chapter 3 ◆ Fluids: when and how to administer them

replacement of the water (rehydration) and electrolytes lost in addition to maintenance fluid therapy. Once the need for resuscitative fluid therapy has been ruled out, the patient's requirements should be assessed before deciding whether a so-called "restrictive" fluid therapy, with a water balance equal to zero, should be provided, or whether fluid therapy should be performed in a liberal manner, that is, infusing generous quantities of fluids. In the former case, restrictive administration of fluids involves replacing those lost using solutions equal in composition and amount to the patient's deficit, while in the latter case, much larger amounts of fluids are administered: for example, in humans, 3–7 L are administered on the day of surgery and more than 3 L per day over the following 3–4 days [9]. These doses correspond to approximately 1.7–4.2 mL/kg/hour on the day of surgery and 1.7 mL/kg/hour on the following days.

Excessive administration of fluids can cause increased blood pressure and hemodilution; it should be remembered that the reduction of hematocrit and viscosity contributes to the collapse of the capillaries and the flow within them [10]; causes tissue and pulmonary edema; reduces the ability to transport oxygen and therefore leads to tissue hypoxia; causes coagulation disorders; increases the blood flow rate, thereby inducing a reduction in the opening in the microcapillaries; and leads to bacterial translocation, increased concentration of atrial natriuretic peptide responsible for glycocalyx damage, sepsis, and delay in wound healing, with an increased risk of dehiscence of surgical sutures. Insufficient fluid administration, on the other hand, can cause other complications, such as insufficient perfusion pressure, reduced oxygen availability (oxygen delivery, DO_2), anaerobic metabolism, hypovolemia, collapse, and possible death of the patient. For these reasons, the administration of fluids must be adapted to the patient's requirements (see Figure 3.1), which can also be estimated based on the hydration and perfusion status.

Hydration

The hydration status is usually assessed through a clinical evaluation, as the methods to calculate the amount of water present in the body require techniques that are not usually accessible in clinical practice (see Chapter 1). Therefore, the interpretation based on clinical parameters is unfortunately subjective and can be altered by factors not dependent on the hydration status, such as obesity or severe slimming and cachexia.

The patient should be weighed during the physical examination, as weight is a useful parameter to establish the volume of fluids to be administered, and then, during fluid therapy, to determine if the patient retains the fluids administered or if there is fluid depletion despite the infusion. The amount of fluid loss is obtained by multiplying the percentage of dehydration, obtained by assessing several physical parameters (Table 3.4), by the body weight expressed in kg; the value obtained corresponds to the liters of fluid to be infused.

Chapter 3 ◆ Fluids: when and how to administer them

Table 3.4 Clinical signs of dehydration

Percentage of dehydration	Clinical signs
5	Undetectable clinical signs
5–6	Dry oral and ocular mucous membranes
6–8	Slight delay in repositioning of skin folds and slight increase in capillary refill time (CRT)
9–12	Severe delay in skin fold repositioning, CRT >2 seconds or absent, dry and hyperemic oral and ocular mucous membranes, sunken eyes, weak pulse and hypotension
>12	Decompensated hypovolemic shock (tachycardia, tachypnea, hypotension, weak pulse, pale mucous membranes, CRT >2 seconds, cold extremities and CNS depression)

For example, if a 15 kg patient shows signs of 10% dehydration, it means that about 1.5 L of fluids should be administered. It is recommended to distribute the volume of fluids to be infused over 24 hours, so as to monitor the evolution of the hydration status and any electrolyte imbalances that may be present. In some cases, for example of severe hypovolemia, the volume of solution necessary to correct dehydration can be infused more quickly (e.g., in 4–12 hours), but careful evaluation is needed of whether fluid resuscitation might be more appropriate than routine fluid therapy.

Calculation of daily fluid therapy

To calculate daily fluid therapy in patients who are unable to drink or who have continuous losses that cannot be replaced by oral administration, the volume of fluids required to replace losses due to dehydration and any other ongoing losses must be added to the maintenance fluids, as shown in the following equation:

$$\text{Daily fluid therapy} = \text{maintenance fluids} + \% \text{ dehydration} + \text{ongoing losses} \qquad (Equation\ 5)$$

"Ongoing losses" means the water and electrolytes lost through vomiting, diarrhea and polyuria, more rarely through sialorrhea or evaporation due to tachypnea that does respond to therapy. Quantification of the ongoing losses is performed by monitoring the output of body fluids, for example through urinary catheterization, or by measuring any fluids collected in a recipient or weighing absorbent materials (e.g.,

Chapter 3 ◆ Fluids: when and how to administer them

hygienic absorbent sleepers) before and after use. Urinary catheterization allows accurate monitoring of the infused fluids and those excreted by the kidneys (*input and output*) and urine production per hour.

For example, a dog weighing 20 kg with 9% dehydration (decrease in skin turgor, CRT of 2.5 seconds and dry oral mucous membranes) and continuous episodes of vomiting (8 episodes/day of about 35 mL each one) will need the following daily fluid therapy:

$$mL/day = (30 \times kg + 70) + (kg \times \% \text{ dehydration}) + (\text{ongoing losses})$$

$$mL/day = (30 \times 20 + 70) + (20 \times 9\%) + (8 \times 35)$$

$$mL/day = 670 + 1800 + 280$$

$$mL/day = 2750$$

$$mL/hour = 114$$

Once lost fluids, calculated on the basis of dehydration, have been replaced (usually after 24 hours), the volume of fluids necessary for rehydration (which in the example corresponds to 1800 mL/day) is subtracted from the total daily fluid volume, and the fluids necessary for maintenance and any ongoing losses are continued until the patient resumes normal eating and the clinical signs disappear. In the example above, if the patient, after 24 hours, is rehydrated and the episodes of vomiting are down to 4 per day, the volume of fluids to be administered in the following 24 hours will be 670 mL + 140 mL, which corresponds to about 34 mL/ hour.

In order to monitor whether the volume of fluids administered meets the patient's needs, it is important to remember that the patient should always be weighed twice a day, so as to reduce the risks of fluid overload or weight loss resulting from insufficient fluid therapy.

To objectively assess whether perfusion and oxygenation are improved thanks to fluid therapy, it is possible to measure $ScvO_2$ (see Table 3.6).

Hemodynamic monitoring

The need to administer fluids to restore effective circulation (i.e., fluid resuscitation) is established by assessing the patient's hemodynamic status using clinical and instrumental examinations. Some of these parameters are static and detect a value at a

Chapter 3 ◆ Fluids: when and how to administer them

particular time, while others are dynamic and therefore allow continuous monitoring of the hemodynamic status.

The *physical perfusion parameters* (Box 3.3) are heart rate, pulse quality, CRT (capillary refill time), mucous membrane color, body temperature, jugular ectasia and urine output.

Heart rate and cardiac output

Heart rate is a parameter that is very simple but very important to measure since it directly affects cardiac output, as expressed in the following equation:

$$CO = SV \times HR \qquad (Equation\ 6)$$

CO, cardiac output; VEF, ventricular ejection fraction; HR, heart rate.

Cardiac output (CO) measures the amount of blood pumped in 1 minute from the left ventricle (see Equation 6); stroke volume (SV) is the volume of blood ejected during each contraction from the left ventricle; heart rate (HR), which is multiplied by the volume of blood ejected during each contraction, can increase or decrease CO. When patients are hypovolemic, the SV is reduced, which causes a reduction in the circulating volume and a rapid response of the body with an increase in heart rate; conversely, a reduction in heart rate can cause a reduction in CO. Therefore, in hemodynamically unstable or hypovolemic patients, attention should be paid to the heart rate, which is usually increased before the fluid bolus and normalizes in patients responsive to fluid therapy. CO can also increase due to increases in myocardial contractility as well as in preload (i.e., the volume of blood that reaches the heart from the venous compartment).

Box 3.3 — **Clinical parameters of perfusion**

- Heart rate: dogs 80–160 bpm; cats and pediatric patients 160–240 bpm
- Pulse: full, hyperdynamic, weak, absent
- Capillary refill time (CRT): 1–2 seconds
- Mucous membrane color: pink, red, pale, yellow, bluish
- Central temperature: rectal or esophageal 38–39 °C
- Peripheral temperature: interdigital 35–36 °C
- Jugular ectasia: evidenced by hemostasis
- Urine output: 1–2 mL/kg/hour

Chapter 3 ♦ Fluids: when and how to administer them

Pulse quality

The peripheral pulse represents the movement of blood on the vascular wall (Figure 3.2). It is an easily detectable, repeatable and useful parameter when evaluating the hemodynamic status, especially when the femoral pulse is compared with the metatarsal pulse (Box 3.4). The pressure wave is transmitted more quickly (about 10 m/s) through the vascular wall, while blood moves at a much lower speed (about 0.5 m/s). Therefore, when the pulse is palpated, more than the movement of blood, what is perceived is the pressure wave moving through the vascular wall.

In critically ill patients, the assessment of pulse quality plays an important role as their condition can change very quickly. In these cases, a rapid and repeatable method that is easily applicable by all medical and paramedical staff can make a difference in the evaluation of the hemodynamic status and response to fluid therapy or inotropes and/or vasopressor drugs, especially when no effective tools are available for this hemodynamic assessment or when these tools fail to provide reliable information and their ability to detect data when the circulation is compromised by excessive vasoconstriction or vasodilation needs to be checked.

The *metatarsal pulse* is the first to disappear (systolic pressure <90 mmHg) during hypovolemia or hypotension; it can be palpated dorsal and medial to the tibiotarsal joint. The femoral pulse becomes absent when systolic pressure becomes severely reduced (<70 mmHg); severe vasoconstriction or vasodilation can also hinder its detection. In addition, a discrepancy between the cardiac auscultation and pulse is a sign of arrhythmia.

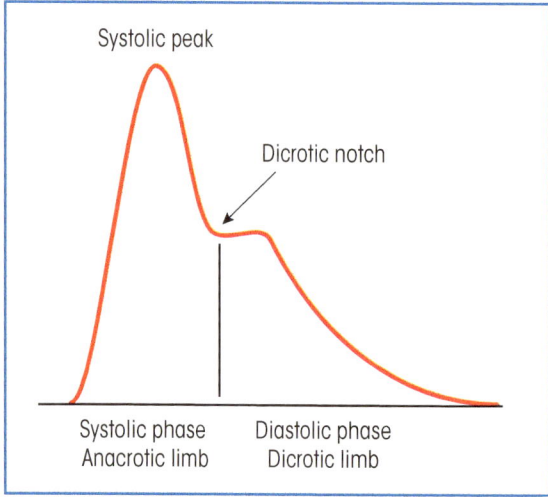

Figure 3.2 Normal pulse, pressure curve.

Chapter 3 ◆ Fluids: when and how to administer them

Box 3.4	Lower empirical pressures at which the pulse cannot be perceived

- Metatarsal pulse: about 90 mmHg
- Femoral pulse: 70 mmHg
- Palpable apical impulse: <50-60 mmHg

In thin patients and particularly in dolichocephalic dogs, the disappearance of a palpable apical impulse on the left chest wall in the cardiac projection area between the third and sixth intercostal spaces may be related to severely impaired myocardial performance, severe hypotension (<50–60 mmHg), and hypoperfusion. When the previously detectable apical impulse disappears, it is necessary to reevaluate the patient, since cardiopulmonary resuscitation or shock fluid therapy may be indispensable.

The peripheral pulse intensity, depth, amplitude, rate, rhythm, length and type should be identified. The peripheral pulse can then be classified as bounding, increased, normal, weak or absent.

Increases in heart rate (>220 bpm) may be suggestive of hypovolemia and tachyarrhythmias; pain can also increase the amplitude of the pulse and reduce its duration, while during decompensated shock the pulse increases in rate but is reduced in amplitude. A weak pulse can be symptomatic of hypovolemia, anemia, or heart failure, while sepsis can generate a hyperkinetic pulse with an increased amplitude, but that disappears easily with digital pressure (i.e., that is very compressible) and with a shorter duration (see Figure 3.2; Figure 3.3). A reduction in duration, amplitude and intensity is typically related to hypovolemia.

Capillary refill time (CRT)

CRT is assessed by causing, with digital pressure, a displacement of the blood from the vascular bed of an accessible mucous membrane (e.g., the gingiva), and then measuring the time necessary for the blood to return to the capillary bed from which it was removed, which is done based on the return of the mucous membrane to its original color. Under normal conditions, the time it takes for the mucous membrane to return to its original color is about 1.5–2 seconds. An increased CRT can be caused by contraction of the precapillary sphincters, capillary vasodilation, and a decreased circulating volume (e.g., hypotension, hypovolemia).

To determine if the CRT is increased due to excessive vasoconstriction or to vasodilation, the temperature of the distal limbs can be assessed by palpation; when vasoconstriction occurs, the temperature of the extremities is decreased and vice versa. It is also possible to measure the rectal and interdigital temperatures with a common

Chapter 3 ◆ Fluids: when and how to administer them

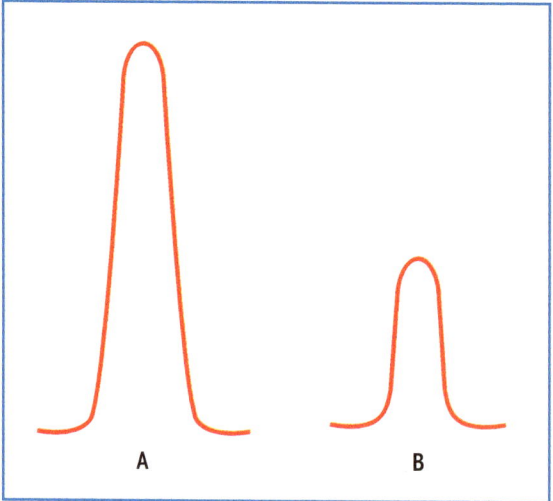

Figure 3.3 **A.** Hyperdynamic pulse. **B.** Hypodynamic pulse.

clinical thermometer. The difference between the rectal and interdigital temperatures, under normal conditions, is about 3–4 °C.

Mucous membrane color

Although it does not always have an unequivocal and pathognomonic interpretation, the color of the mucous membranes is important to recognize signs of pathological processes that are not always readily diagnosed. The mucous membranes can be injected or bright red in case of sepsis and septic shock; red, hyperemic, in case of hyperthermia, hypertension, vasodilation, intoxication, hyperthyroidism; pale, in case of anemia, vasoconstriction, hypotension, hypovolemic shock; bluish, in case of hypoxemia, cyanosis; brown, in case of methemoglobinemia; yellow, in case of jaundice, severe hepatic insufficiency, administration of hemoglobin glutamer; and grayish, in case of severe oxygen deficiency, decompensated shock, imminent death.

Body temperature

Body temperature plays a very important role in critically ill patients, and a decreased temperature can be a suggestive sign of reduced activity of the central nervous system (CNS). Severe hypothermia can be a sign of imminent cardiopulmonary arrest because the thermoregulatory center is located near the cardiorespiratory center.

Chapter 3 ◆ Fluids: when and how to administer them

A reduction in body temperature can affect many vital functions, such as coagulation and the acid–base balance. In critically ill human patients, a body temperature below 32 °C is related to 100% mortality. For this reason, an attempt must always be made in critically ill patients to correct hypothermia with active or passive systems.

Active systems are devices capable of generating heat, such as hot air devices, which are effective as they heat the patient evenly without placing them in contact with hot surfaces that could cause exemia due to vasodilation and therefore aggravate an already compromised circulation; systems that use semiconductive fabrics (e.g., Hot Dog®), which provide heating of the patient by direct contact; infrared lamps and electric mats, which can however cause second- to third-degree burns in addition to plasmatic exemia if they are not used appropriately.

Passive systems are suitable to avoid heat dispersion at the body surface; for this purpose, thermal blankets (e.g., wool) or aluminum blankets may be used. Passive systems are used when heat loss must be avoided in mild hypothermia, while active systems are used in severe forms of hypothermia, because they are able to generate heat.

Body temperature should be measured centrally, when possible, by inserting a temperature probe in the esophagus at the level of the base of the heart; a simpler technique is to measure it rectally with a clinical thermometer. The interdigital temperature can be measured using a common clinical thermometer or with the temperature probe of a multiparameter monitor. The interdigital temperature is useful to for comparison with the central temperature: a reduction >3–4 °C is suggestive of peripheral vasoconstriction and therefore of a circulatory alteration capable of hindering peripheral and organ perfusion.

Jugular vein distension

Jugular vein distension can be detected at the level of the jugular fossa on the side of the neck. To identify it, an area of about 15 x 5 cm should be clipped along an imaginary line that runs from the corner of the jaw to the tip of the shoulder. To cause ectasia of the jugular vein, hemostasis is achieved by exerting pressure with two fingers at the level of the entrance of the jugular vein into the chest, at the medial surface of the shoulder tip. Under normal conditions it is most evident after 3–4 seconds and disappears within 1–2 seconds. The absence of ectasia despite exerting pressure on the vein indicates hypovolemia of the venous compartment or severe heart failure, while ectasia with no hemostasis indicates an excess of blood volume in the venous compartment; a jugular pulse may be due to right cardiac regurgitation, an increase in intrathoracic pressure (e.g., effusion or pneumothorax), or a pericardial effusion.

Chapter 3 ◆ Fluids: when and how to administer them

Urine production

Urine production is a useful parameter to determine whether the body is able to eliminate the catabolites of metabolism and some trace elements and to maintain the water, electrolyte and acid–base balance. A reduction in urine production in a normohydrated patient can be considered an indication of impaired perfusion, as the kidneys receive about 25% of cardiac output. Arterial pressures <70 mmHg may be responsible for impaired renal perfusion, as the kidney is able to regulate perfusion when the blood pressure is between 70 and 200 mmHg; hypotension therefore causes a reduction in renal blood flow (RBF) and urine output.

Under normal conditions, urine output should be about 1–2 mL/kg/hour. Small patients have a higher urine production than large ones.

If the composition of the urine does not reflect the ongoing pathological process, then another unidentified pathological process may be present, or the kidneys may be damaged. If renal function is normal and excess fluids are administered, the compensation will be an increase in urine output; conversely, in case of dehydration, the kidneys will concentrate urine.

This is why, in a dehydrated patient, the urine should be more concentrated (increased specific gravity). If a dehydrated patient's urine has a low specific gravity or there is oliguria in the presence of systemic or pulmonary edema, the renal function should be assessed as it is likely to be compromised.

Parameters to evaluate the hemodynamic status

The instrumental parameters to assess a patient's hemodynamic status can be static or dynamic. Dynamic parameters are most effective in assessing a patient's response to fluid therapy. The use of dynamic parameters allows the implementation of the so-called goal-directed therapy (GDT). It is not possible to determine if the objectives of fluid therapy have been achieved and if the patient is responsive to fluid resuscitation with static parameters (Box 3.5). Not all hemodynamic instrumental parameters can assess whether the patient will respond to the fluid bolus (*fluid responder*), and unfortunately most of these parameters have only been evaluated in human patients, so their reliability and the normal values in our patients have not yet been determined. The parameters that can identify *fluid responders* are: clinical parameters detected at regular intervals, SVV, PPV, SPV, PVI, cardiac ouput with esophageal Doppler, inferior vena cava diameter (IVCD) variation, CVCCI and end-expiratory occlusion (see Chapter 1).

Blood pressure (BP)

BP is the measurement of the pulsatile pressure wave that moves from the aortic valve to the arteries. During systole, BP increases and is called systolic blood pres-

Chapter 3 ◆ Fluids: when and how to administer them

> **Box 3.5 — Static and dynamic parameters for hemodynamic assessment**
>
> **Static parameters**
> - Invasive or non-invasive blood pressure: MAP >70 mmHg or systolic ≥90 mmHg.
> - $ScvO_2$: 70%.
> - CVP (central venous pressure), normal values: 0–5 cmH_2O; circulatory overload: >10 cmH_2O.
> - PCWP (pulmonary capillary wedge pressure): pulmonary artery catheter needed (Swan–Ganz catheter).
> - Chest X-ray, e.g., pulmonary edema, hypovolemic condition with microcardia, hypervolemia.
>
> **Dynamic parameters**
> - CVC (caudal vena cava): diameter variation during breathing.
> - Echocardiography.
> - Clinical evaluation: of limited value, but can detect inadequate organ perfusion if repeated frequently.
> - Esophageal Doppler: requires general anesthesia and specific instrument.
> - SVV (stroke volume variation): requires controlled positive pressure ventilation and veterinary validation.
> - End-expiratory occlusion test: requires controlled positive pressure ventilation and veterinary validation.
> - PPV (pulse pressure variation) >10%: requires controlled positive pressure ventilation and veterinary validation.
> - PVI (pulse variation index) >14%: requires controlled positive pressure ventilation and veterinary validation.

sure, while during diastole it decreases and is called diastolic blood pressure. The arterial pressure waveform has two distinct parts, an ascending anacrotic limb and a descending dicrotic limb. The steepness of the wave is related to myocardial contractility; closure of the aortic valve is responsible for a short deceleration of the blood flow that corresponds to the dicrotic notch (see Figure 3.2).

BP measures the hydrostatic pressure of arterial blood; it is therefore an important parameter to evaluate whether the blood can reach peripheral circulation and thus ensure effective peripheral perfusion. Peripheral vasoconstriction, which causes an increase in systemic vascular resistance (SVR), hinders organ and peripheral perfusion, but it can compensate for the reduced circulating volume and keep BP within normal or close to normal values. For these reasons, BP alone cannot be considered as a parameter of organ or peripheral perfusion, even if it may be impaired by severe hypotension. Peripheral vasodilation can also occur as a compensatory mechanism for the increase in CO, as occurs for example during a physical activity that increases heart rate. Both a persistent reduction and an increase in BP can cause organ failure, in particular of the kidneys, CNS, eyeballs and heart.

Chapter 3 ◆ Fluids: when and how to administer them

The most common causes of hypertension are hypervolemia, the use of vasoconstrictor drugs (e.g., sympathomimetic amines) or drugs responsible for water retention (e.g., corticosteroids, nonsteroidal anti-inflammatory drugs, salt, estrogens, antidepressant drugs, progestins, and finasteride). The pathological processes that may be responsible for water retention are renal failure, liver failure, diabetes mellitus, hypothyroidism, hypoadrenocorticism, congestive heart failure, and hyperadrenocorticism. The pathological processes that can cause hypotension are hypovolemia, dehydration, sepsis, septic shock, distributive shock, cardiogenic shock, and vasodilation.

The mean arterial pressure (MAP) must be between 50 and 150 mmHg to ensure adequate cerebral blood flow (CBF), so in patients with head trauma, monitoring of systemic BP is a fundamental parameter to control secondary damage to the brain and spinal tissue (Figure 3.4, Table 3.5). BP can be measured both noninvasively (NIBP, noninvasive blood pressure) or invasively (IBP, invasive blood pressure). The first method, which is the most widely used, can be performed more easily and quickly than IBP measurement.

Noninvasive blood pressure (NIBP)

Unfortunately, NIBP can provide unreliable data because it is obtained through an inflatable cuff (Figure 3.5) placed around the extremity of a limb or at the base of the tail, and so is affected by tremors of the skeletal muscles of the limbs, peripheral vasoconstriction, tachycardia, and arrhythmias. NIBP generally overestimates low pressures and underestimates high pressures.

Cuffs not appropriate to the patient's size can alter the measurement: cuffs that are too wide can give falsely reduced measurements, while cuffs that are too narrow can produce falsely increased measurements. Therefore, when taking measurements, it is recommended to record the size of the cuff used, so as to always use the same for that patient. The inflatable cuff must be adapted to the diameter of the limb or tail; its length must be about 80% of that of the limb and its width 40% of the circumference of the limb.

To reduce artifacts produced by tremors, it is recommended to place the cuff around the base of the tail. This site is better tolerated in awake patients than the limbs, especially in trauma cases in which the limbs may not be a suitable site for measurement and constriction by the inflatable cuff could cause intolerance reactions, in particular if the patient is suffering from acute pain. The limbs, at the level of the humerus or, worse, the femur, have a conical longitudinal section that hinders the correct positioning of the inflatable cuff, which thus affects measurements. For this reason, it is advisable to wrap the cuff around the second distal third of the forelimb, with the cuff tube in a position corresponding to that of the artery.

When the cuff is wrapped around the base of the tail, the hair on its ventral aspect should be clipped in the case of patients with long hair (e.g., Persian cat or Maltese

Chapter 3 ◆ Fluids: when and how to administer them

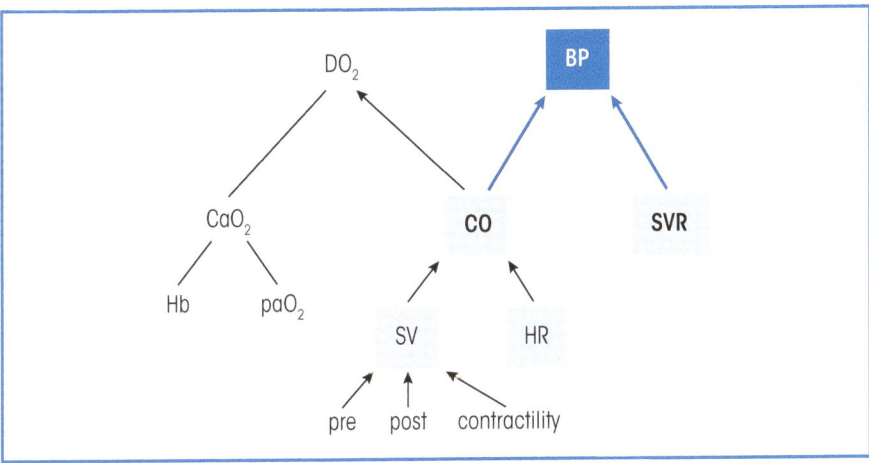

Figure 3.4 Components of DO_2 and blood pressure. BP, blood pressure; CaO_2, total oxygen content; CO, cardiac output; DO_2, availability of oxygen; Hb, hemoglobin; HR, heart rate; paO_2, partial oxygen pressure; pre, preload; post, afterload; SV, stroke volume; SVR, systemic vascular resistance.

Table 3.5 Normal blood pressure values

Parameter	Dog	Cat
SAP	90–150	85–160
DAP	60–90	60–90
MAP	70–100	70–110

DAP, diastolic blood pressure; MAP, mean blood pressure; SAP, systolic blood pressure.

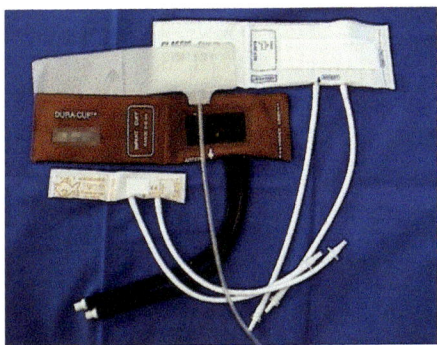

Figure 3.5 Inflatable cuff for measuring blood pressure.

Chapter 3 ◆ Fluids: when and how to administer them

dog) so that the variation in the arterial wall diameter is more easily picked up by the instrument performing the oscillometric measurement. The position of the cuff tube for measurements at the base of the tail should also correspond to that of the caudal artery (ventral and medial).

Mean arterial pressure (MAP)

Once NIBP has been measured, it is possible, using a mathematical calculation, to obtain the MAP. The systolic phase constitutes about 1/3 of the entire cardiac cycle, while the diastolic phase constitutes about 2/3 of the cardiac cycle; this is why, when calculating the MAP, the SAP is divided by three, as in the following formula:

$$MAP = DAP + (SAP - DAP)/3 \qquad \text{(Equation 7)}$$

MAP, mean arterial pressure; DAP, diastolic blood pressure; SAP, systolic blood pressure.

In the presence of tachycardia this time interval is altered and the MAP is affected, while under normal conditions the MAP is closer to organ perfusion pressure. For these reasons, peripheral perfusion is not only influenced by DAP, but also by the difference between SAP and DAP. To obtain a peripheral perfusion pressure capable of supporting the vital functions of tissues and therefore of the organ, the MAP should be at least 70 mmHg. Normal values in dogs and cats are given in Tables 3.6 and 3.7. Thanks to SVR self-regulation mechanisms, the brain can maintain organ perfusion for MAP values between 50–150 mmHg, while the kidneys need a slightly higher ideal pressure of 70–200 mmHg.

Doppler ultrasonic method

The Doppler ultrasonic method to measure NIBP requires an instrument capable of generating 10 MHz ultrasound waves, which detect the passage of blood through the peripheral arteries and, in exotic patients, also through the heart chambers or large vessels.

To take the measurement, the probe of the instrument is applied at the level of the common palmar digital artery of the hindlimb or frontlimb, after placing ultrasound gel between the patient's skin and the surface of the probe to prevent the presence of air bubbles from hindering the passage of ultrasound. The area above the artery must therefore be clipped, as would be done in preparation for surgery. The chosen area does not require surgical preparation. The probe is attached to the limb with the help of an adhesive plaster.

The flow of red blood cells inside the vessel is responsible for the variations detected by the probe. These are then conducted to the instrument, which generates the typical sound. The intensity of the sound produced depends on the blood flow in the vessel: the greater the blood flow, the greater the intensity of the sound.

Chapter 3 ◆ Fluids: when and how to administer them

Table 3.6 Objectives of fluid therapy

Parameter	Normal goals	Minimum goals

Heart rate
  Dog
  Cat
	80–160 bpm
	>160 <240 bpm
		80–140 bpm
		200–240 bpm

Pulse	Full	Palpable
CRT	<2 seconds	<2 seconds
Color of mucous membranes	pink	pink
Rectal temperature Extremity temperature	37.5–38.0 °C 34.5 °C	36.0 °C 33.0 °C
Mean blood pressure	≥70 mmHg	≥60 mmHg
Urine output	1–2 mL/kg/hour	0.5 mL/kg/hour
Lactate	<2.5 mmol/L	2.5–3.5 mmol/L
$ScvO_2$	>70%	>70%

Normal goals: hypovolemia, severe dehydration; minimum goals: ongoing active hemorrhage, pulmonary and cerebral edema, coagulopathies.

Table 3.7 Shock: consequences and therapy

Shock	Physiopathology	Preload	CO	SVR	SVR
Hypovolemic	Hemorrhage or reduction ECF and ICF	↓↓	↓	↑	Fluids
Distributive	Sepsis, septic shock, GDV, pancreatitis, vasodilation, SVR, systemic inflammation	↓↓	↑↓	↓↓	Vasoactive amines (e.g., norepinephrine)
Cardiogenic	DCM, HCM, CCF, cardiac hypertrophy, cardiac tamponade, mediastinal diseases, toxins, medications	↑↓	↓↓	↑	Etiological therapy (e.g., dobutamine, oxygen, chest drainage)

CO, cardiac output; DCM, dilated cardiomyopathy of dog; HCM, feline hypertrophic cardiomyopathy; GDV, gastric dilatation volvulus; CCF, congestive cardiac failure; SVR, systemic vascular resistance.

Chapter 3 ◆ Fluids: when and how to administer them

Once the probe has been placed, an inflatable cuff with the characteristics (length and width) described above must be placed upstream of the probe. The cuff is inflated until the sound generated by the instrument disappears; it is then slowly deflated. Systolic pressure is the value obtained when the first audible sound appears. About 15 mmHg are added to this value since this method slightly underestimates the peak pressure. Unfortunately, it is not possible to determine the DAP with a sufficient objective approximation, as it would correspond to the variation in intensity of the sound emitted during the continuous deflation of the cuff after the appearance of the first audible sound.

This method is very useful when wanting to know the peripheral perfusion of a particular region (intensity of the sound produced by the Doppler device); for example, the common palmar digital arteries can be used to assess peripheral perfusion, or the probe can be applied to the corneal surface (where ultrasound gel was previously placed) during cardiocirculatory resuscitation to check if resuscitation maneuvers are able to restore cerebral blood flow. Continuous and intense sounds indicate good perfusion, while weak or absent sounds are suggestive of poor perfusion. The Doppler ultrasound method offers the following advantages: it assesses local perfusion, it can measure SAP even in very small and hypotensive patients, it detects the pulse when this cannot be done by digital pressure, and it enables assessment of the presence of peripheral vasoconstriction or vasodilation as well as its duration based on the intensity of the sound emitted (e.g., during general anesthesia, hypotension produced by vasodilation by drugs is responsible for a reduction in sound intensity). Reduction of the pulse quality may be useful when checking for an increase in intrathoracic pressure (e.g., pneumothorax).

The main disadvantages of the method are that it can only measure the SAP; an operator is needed to perform the procedure; BP measurements cannot be obtained at predetermined intervals; the method is poorly tolerated by awake patients, especially in the feline species and in patients in pain; the procedure is difficult to perform in hypotensive and vasoconstricted patients; and detection is operator-dependent, since the first sound corresponding to the SAP may be detected differently by different operators.

Invasive blood pressure (IBP) measurement

Invasive blood pressure (IBP) measurement is the best technique for assessing blood pressure, because it directly determines the blood pressure in a peripheral or central arterial vessel. The change in blood pressure inside the vessel is transformed into an electric signal thanks to a transducer, which sends the signal to a monitor that amplifies it and generates a graphical representation of the pressure waves. It is not affected by the artifacts that affect NIBP, such as vasoconstriction, hypotension, hypertension, and arrhythmias, but requires catheterization of an artery. The same

Chapter 3 ◆ Fluids: when and how to administer them

arterial access used for IBP can also be used to collect serial arterial samples for performing a blood gas analysis to monitor cardiorespiratory function. Typically, this catheter is placed in the dorsal metatarsal artery (Figure 3.6), but the coccygeal and radial arteries can also be used. In very small patients, it is necessary to use arteries of a larger diameter, such as the femoral artery.

Changes in blood pressure are comparable in most arteries because blood is a noncompressible liquid and spreads the sphygmic wave in the various arterial districts to a comparable degree. The pressure will remain undetected or be unreliable only in the case of local circulatory impairment or in the presence of clots or a bent catheter. The chosen artery should be identified with the index finger; the area is then surgically prepared and a 21–23 gauge IV catheter is flushed with heparinized saline (e.g., normal saline containing 1 IU of heparin sodium/mL), before inserting the IV catheter through the skin at an angle of about 15–30°, in the opposite direction to blood flow. The catheter can remain in situ for 5–7 days. If inflammation or swelling appears near the IV catheter insertion site, it should be removed and the site of insertion changed. To avoid tissue ischemia from obstruction of the vessel, the IV catheter patency and local peripheral perfusion should be monitored at least every 8 hours, along with the interdigital temperature (which must be about 3–4 °C lower than the rectal temperature) and, when possible, the skin color.

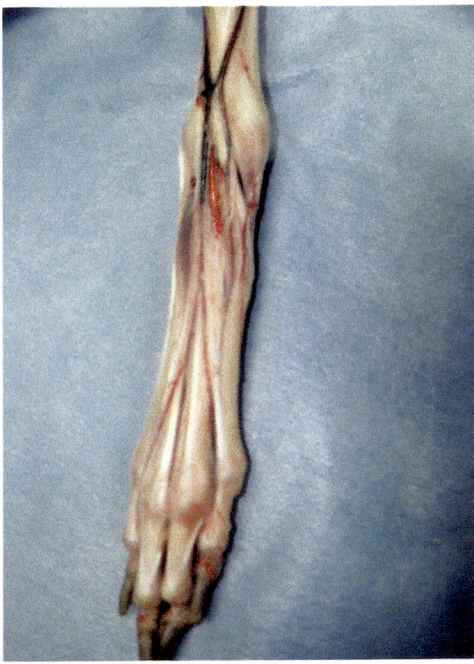

Figure 3.6 Metatarsal artery.

Chapter 3 ♦ Fluids: when and how to administer them

Technique

Once the IV catheter has been inserted into the vessel and as soon as blood appears, the needle is withdrawn while at the same time continuing to fully insert the catheter into the artery. The IV catheter should be secured in place with adhesive tape and connected to an extension tube equipped with a three-way stopcock, previously filled with heparinized saline; the three-way stopcock is connected to the pressure transducer, which must be placed at the height of the patient's right atrium.

The transducer is equipped with a diaphragm: when the blood, thanks to the thrust received from the heart and mostly to the elasticity of the large vessels, hits the diaphragm, it causes its distension. This displacement is then converted into an electrical impulse, which the monitor amplifies (through an amplifier) and shows on the device's screen.

An IV line connected to a bag of heparinized saline is connected to the perpendicular port of the three-way stopcock (in a vertical position with respect to the IV catheter). Then (using an electric cable provided in the kit) the transducer is connected to the monitor, the bag containing saline solution is compressed using a pressure bag (300 mmHg), and any air bubbles that might be present in the circuit is removed, thus creating a pressure greater than the patient's systolic pressure.

Subsequently, the monitor is zeroed by opening the transducer to the environment to neutralize the effect of atmospheric pressure (760 mmHg at sea level) and setting this pressure value as zero. At this point, the patient is connected to the monitor through the three-way stopcock to start arterial blood pressure measurements. The device should be zeroed every 8 hours, or whenever the patient is mobilized or their decubitus changed, or when measurements are doubtful. The infusion rate should be approximately 3mL/hour; the resonance frequency (distance between two systolic peaks divided by the velocity) should be greater than 30 Hz when the patient has an HR ≥180 bpm and >20 Hz for an HR of up to 120 bpm.

Indications and interpretation

IBP measurement is particularly indicated if continuous monitoring of BP over an entire cardiac cycle needs to be performed, in the presence of vasoconstriction, or in patients with or at risk of severe hypotension that could compromise vital functions and cause death. Some typical cases of hypotension that benefit from continuous monitoring of IBP are sepsis, septic shock, general anesthesia (especially with gaseous anesthetic agents) in high-risk patients, when vasoactive amines are administered to evaluate their effectiveness, during a fluid challenge test to evaluate the efficacy and duration of effect of the bolus, and when deciding whether vasoactive amines need to be administered because fluid boluses are not effective.

In addition to providing numerical data concerning arterial pressures, IBP measurement makes it possible, through the study of the sphygmic wave, to evaluate

Chapter 3 ◆ Fluids: when and how to administer them

myocardial contractility, the transmission of the pressure wave through the vascular wall, and blood flow dynamics. The first phase of the waveform, called anacrotic limb, shows a rapid increase that reaches a peak called systolic or anacrotic peak (under normal conditions, in dogs it is about 90–150 mmHg). The beginning of the first phase coincides with the contraction of the left ventricle, the opening of the aortic valve, and the outflow of blood from the ventricle, which generates a pressure wave on the wall of the aortic root that is then transmitted to all the arteries. The inclination, or rather the steepness, of the anacrotic limb and its height depend on the speed of the blood, and they are an expression of the contractility and function of the left ventricle. The steepness increases in hypervolemic patients or when cardiac inotropy increases, while it is reduced in hypovolemic patients, when cardiac contractility is reduced (e.g., due to dilated cardiomyopathy), or when both situations occur. The peak of the waveform becomes more acute in hypovolemic patients or when a reduction in CO occurs.

The dicrotic notch corresponds to the closure of the aortic valve, when the wave starts to rapidly decrease to reach zero at the end of systole. The effect of the wall of vessels with a lower diameter than that of the aorta can sometimes cause undulations that can be detected along the dicrotic limb. In elderly patients, as ventricular contractility becomes less effective and arterial stiffening increases, the waveform may decrease in height, and the anacrotic and dicrotic limbs may become less steep (the curve flattens and widens).

Vasodilation causes a reduction in the peak as well as rounding of the waveform, hypovolemia leads to a reduction in the peak and amplitude of the waveform, and hypotension causes the disappearance of the peak (tip shape) and dicrotic notch. Conversely, vasoconstriction can cause an increase in the peak, while arrhythmias typically reduce the ventricular filling volume, which increases the steepness of the anacrotic limb and a reduction in the peak.

Pressure waveforms are a complex set of oscillatory waves that have a particular frequency and amplitude. Together they constitute the classic sphygmic wave that is observed on the monitor and is called harmonic frequency. The monitor detects harmonic frequencies at each pulse and shows them on the screen with the typical shape (see Figure 3.4). *Underdamping* refers to an exaggerated response due to the alteration of the harmonic frequency that occurs when the tube is too soft and too long or during tachydysrhytmias. This phenomenon shows an increase of the systolic pressure characterized by a narrow systolic peak and oscillation of the dicrotic limb causing an overestimation of the systolic pressure and an understimation of the diastolic pressure. Conversely, *overdamping* refers to an attenuated response due to the alteration of the harmonic frequency that occurs if the tube is too long (>1 m), if it is too soft, if the arterial catheter is too small, or if air bubbles are present. In case of overdamping the wave is flatter with a reduced or absent dicrotic wave.

Chapter 3 ◆ Fluids: when and how to administer them

Measurement of lactatemia

The measurement of lactatemia has gained a lot of attention in recent years following the development of guidelines for the management of severe sepsis and septic shock by the Surviving Sepsis Campaign in 2016; these suggest, among other objectives of resuscitation, normalizing lactate levels in patients with hyperlactatemia (grade 2C recommendation).

Lactate is a molecule that consists of three carbon atoms and a carboxyl group capable of accepting a hydrogen ion and producing lactic acid. Lactate is synthesized in the cytoplasm of cells due to the presence of lactate dehydrogenase (LDH), which allows the conversion of pyruvate and the regeneration of NAD$^+$ (nicotinamide adenine dinucleotide), as shown in the following equation:

$$CH_3COCOO^- \text{ (pyruvate)} + NADH \leftrightarrow CH_3CHOHCOO^- \text{ (lactate)} + NAD^+ + H^+$$

(Equation 8)

NADH and ATP are produced in sufficient amounts only under aerobic conditions. NADH is needed to convert pyruvate into lactate. The greater the availability of NADH, the greater the production of pyruvate, which enters the Krebs cycle as acetyl-coenzyme A to produce energy, CO_2 and water. Under anaerobic conditions, lactate cannot be oxidized to pyruvate, so its concentration increases (the equilibrium shifts to the right, see Equation 8). If lactate is not oxidized it will also produce an increase in the hydrogen ion concentration (the equilibrium shifts to the right, see Equation 8). Lactate metabolism therefore requires mitochondrial aerobic metabolism; when this cannot happen, an increase in lactatemia occurs. Lactatemia can also increase due to an enzyme deficit responsible for a lack of pyruvate dehydrogenase, which converts pyruvate into acetyl-coenzyme A, or due to causes other than anaerobiosis, which induce the so-called type B lactatemia, such as diabetes mellitus, hypoglycemia, liver disease, systemic neoplasms, sepsis, renal failure, salicylate intoxication, carbon monoxide inhalation, ethylene glycol poisoning, administration of albuterol, or hereditary diseases (mitochondrial myopathy, gluconeogenesis deficiency).

After ruling out the presence of type B hyperlactatemia, it is necessary to check whether the patient's increase in lactate results from a pathology able to cause a release of catecholamines and alter the perfusion and oxygenation of tissues, or if there is an increased demand for oxygen that is not satisfied by oxygenation and tissue perfusion. This condition is called type A hyperlactatemia. Some examples are sepsis, shock, septic shock, congestive heart failure, systolic heart failure, cardiopulmonary arrest, pulmonary edema, seizure, and exercise.

Chapter 3 ◆ Fluids: when and how to administer them

The production of lactate ensures the synthesis of two molecules of ATP instead of the 36 produced by 1 mole of glucose during aerobic metabolism; in addition, two protons are consumed for the synthesis of lactate, so the production of lactate does not cause metabolic acidosis, but actually delays it. Except for type B hyperlactatemia, hyperlactatemia is not a disease in itself but a marker of perfusion. An ineffective tissue perfusion is one of the causes of increased lactatemia [11]. Hypoxia alone is not responsible for an increase in lactatemia, as demonstrated in a study conducted in healthy men who were climbing Mount Everest, in which a median lactatemia of 2.2 mmol/L was found, even with a paO_2 of 25 mmHg [12]. The major organs producing lactate are the skeletal muscles, intestines, brain, erythrocytes, and skin. Lactate is used for gluconeogenesis mainly by the liver and kidneys, and as fuel mostly by the brain and myocardium, which rely on its oxidation for energy production, especially under conditions of stress.

During sepsis, hyperlactatemia derives, rather than from a deficit of tissue perfusion and oxygenation, from an increase in production due to stress, which generates an adrenergic stimulation that produces energy by oxidizing lactate [13]. During hyperlactatemia, the myocardium uses lactate as an energy source for more than half of its energy needs. For these reasons, an increased lactatemia should not be considered as a negative fact, but as the marker of a type of metabolic activity that allows the body to survive stress.

Ringer's lactate solution does not cause lactic acidosis, because it is transformed into a buffer in the liver, but it can alter the measurement of lactate concentration if the blood sample is collected shortly after its administration. Normal lactate values are approximately 2.5 mmol/L. A description of the methods for measuring the other hemodynamic parameters and of how to interpret them is given in Chapter 1.

Fluid resuscitation

So-called fluid responders who require fluid resuscitation are typically patients suffering from hypovolemic or traumatic shock. In the first case, these patients have ineffective tissue perfusion due to a reduction in the circulating blood volume caused by fluid losses from the extracellular and/or intracellular space (e.g., vomiting, diarrhea, and polyuria). These patients are those who respond best to fluid therapy.

Patients with an insufficient circulating blood volume and ineffective organ perfusion due to traumatic shock may be hypovolemic as a result of a rapid blood loss of more than 20–30% of the total circulating volume, or because the site of trauma has caused the release of vasoactive and myocardial depressing agents, which may be

Chapter 3 ♦ Fluids: when and how to administer them

responsible for a circulatory failure resulting from an increase in blood vessel capacitance of both the venous and arterial compartments.

In the latter case, fluid resuscitation cannot restore an adequate systemic circulation and can in fact aggravate the patient's condition, because the administration of large volumes of fluids over a short period of time can cause tissue edema, especially in the presence of prerenal failure caused by prolonged hypotension.

Before administering several fluid boluses, it is necessary to check that the patient does not have an increased venous or arterial capacitance or both. This manifests as vasodilation (e.g., hot extremities) and reduced SVR. The clinical history helps to identify these patients.

The pathological processes that can cause vasodilation are sepsis, septic shock, pancreatitis, trauma, systemic inflammation, systemic neoplasms, heat stroke, burns, autoimmune diseases, ischemic diseases, some snake poisons, and inflammatory gastroenteric diseases. Hypovolemic patients who need fluid resuscitation may show the following signs: tachycardia, prolonged CTR, hypotension, hypothermia, cold extremities, and dry mucous membranes.

Patients responsive to fluid therapy can be identified by monitoring hemodynamic parameters after the administration of a fluid bolus. The evaluation of hemodynamic parameters can be clinical (see above) or instrumental (see Chapter 1) [14].

The instrumentally measured hemodynamic parameters used in humans to identify patients who respond to fluid therapy are still a subject of controversy; some of these are SVV, PPV, end-expiratory occlusion maneuver, and CO measured with esophageal Doppler and other methods (see Chapter 1).

Goal-directed therapy

Fluid therapy aimed at optimizing the hemodynamic status, also known as GDT (goal-directed therapy), began to be used in the 1980s when, with the use of the thermodilution pulmonary artery catheter (Swan–Ganz catheter), it became possible to measure the PAOP (pulmonary artery occlusion pressure). With the Swan–Ganz catheter, CO measurement also became possible and, in 1988, W. Shoemaker [15] published the first study that showed how an increase in DO_2 (measured by placing a Swan–Ganz catheter and determining the CO) led to a reduction in mortality in high-risk surgical patients. To do so, a therapeutic protocol was used that increased DO_2 through the administration of fluids, inotropic drugs (mainly dobutamine) and vasoactive amines; this laid the foundations for other protocols for the management of critically ill patients still in use today. The goal of GDT is to treat hypovolemia, hypoxia, and decreased blood flow. The Swan-Ganz catheter was then abandoned due to the side effects of such invasive monitoring and the introduction of other less invasive monitoring methods that measured CO, such as SVV, PPV, esophageal Dop-

Chapter 3 ◆ Fluids: when and how to administer them

pler, LiDCO and plethysmographic variability index (see Chapter 1). The scientific literature, however, reports contradictory data. For example, a systematic review by the Cochrane Library, which evaluated 31 studies involving 5292 human patients [16], found that GDT—through the administration of fluids, associated when necessary with inotropic and vasoactive drugs, and the consequent increase in DO_2 and improvement of systemic blood flow—does not reduce mortality, but decreases morbidity (hospital stay 1 day shorter, but no reduction in the length of stay in the intensive care unit) of renal and respiratory complications and wound healing time. However, for nine other causes of morbidity (arrhythmias, pneumonia, sepsis, abdominal or urinary infections, myocardial infarction, congestive heart failure, pulmonary edema, and deep thrombosis), no improvements were achieved. The parameters used to perform GDT were the cardiac index (CI, which is obtained by dividing the CO by the body surface area), DO_2, oxygen consumption (VO_2), SV and the parameters derived from it (e.g., SVV), central venous oxygen saturation ($ScvO_2$), oxygen extraction ratio (O_2ER), and lactatemia.

Another randomized multicenter study conducted in 734 patients [17] concluded that GDT does not reduce mortality at 30 days postsurgery but reduces complications in patients undergoing gastrointestinal surgery.

The analysis of these studies shows that critical human patients at higher risk of mortality could benefit from invasive monitoring of hemodynamic parameters, such as CO and SVV; in veterinary medicine, the same benefits could be obtained by noninvasive monitoring of parameters such as PPV, lactatemia and the variation in the diameter of the vena cava. Nonhypovolemic patients with a reduced risk of mortality could benefit from a more restrictive daily fluid therapy with a zero balance.

Hypovolemic dogs and cats showing alterations of perfusion parameters, such as hypotension, increased CTR, reduced CO, reduced urine output, or increased azotemia and lactatemia, or those with impaired blood flow and oxygenation detected by the methods described above, require rapid normalization of these parameters (see Tables 3.6 and 3.7). In patients receiving fluid resuscitation, instrumental monitoring of the following parameters should be performed: MAP, CVP, CO or SVV, SpO_2, lactatemia or $ScvO_2$, and urine output.

Crystalloids or colloids?

The fluids used to restore an effective circulating blood volume are crystalloids and colloids (Figure 3.7). Which are most effective has not yet been demonstrated, although a recent multicenter and randomized study [18] conducted in human patients concluded that colloid fluid resuscitation of critically ill patients at risk of death from trauma, burns, or surgery does not reduce the risk of death, which is even increased if hydroxyethyl starch is used. Finally, given the higher cost of colloids compared to crystalloids, no reason has emerged to prefer the former to the latter.

Chapter 3 ◆ Fluids: when and how to administer them

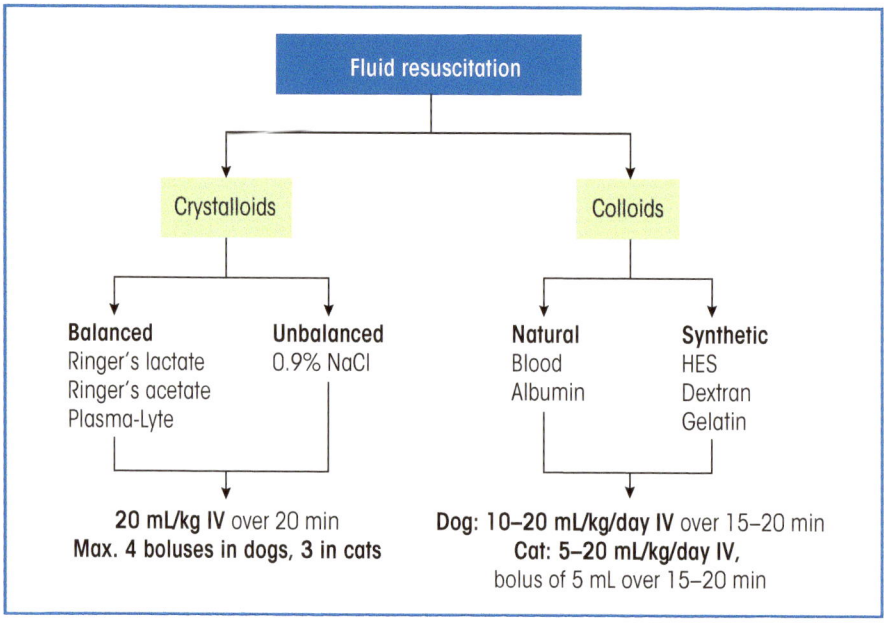

Figure 3.7 Fluid resuscitation. HES, hydroxyethyl starch; Plasma-Lyte, electrolyte replacement solution with sodium gluconate.

Another recent randomized study [19] conducted in 2305 human patients, which evaluated fluid resuscitation with colloids vs. with crystalloids in critically ill patients admitted to intensive care and in a state of hypovolemic shock, found mortality to be similar at 28 days, but reduced with crystalloids at 90 days. The authors considered this conclusion as tentative and pointed out that further confirmation is needed regarding the efficacy described.

In veterinary medicine there is no evidence of such an effect [20]. According to two studies [21,22] it seems that damage to renal function is more present when hydroxyethyl starch (HES) is used at high concentrations (10% HES is more harmful than tetrastarch at 6%). According to the revision of Starling's law (see Chapter 1), when capillary pressure is low, infused crystalloids should remain in the circulation as much as colloidal solutions. This is supported by a human study [23] that showed that crystalloids seem to be more effective in restoring blood plasma volume when infused during anesthesia after trauma than when administered in healthy patients in experimental studies, because renal *clearance* in these conditions is only 10–20%. Therefore, considering the evidence gathered in human medicine, the lack of randomized multicenter studies in veterinary medicine and the absence of evidence, in

Chapter 3 ◆ Fluids: when and how to administer them

dogs and cats, of a greater effectiveness of colloid solutions compared to crystalloids, fluid resuscitation usually consists in the administration of crystalloid boluses until the targeted objectives are achieved.

The type of crystalloid to be used in resuscitation depends on the patient's needs (acid–base balance [SID] and electrolytes [at least sodium, potassium, and chloride]). In the absence of these data, the use of balanced crystalloid solutions is recommended. If invasive parameters cannot be used to monitor the effectiveness of fluid administration in hypovolemic patients (fluid responsiveness), as is done, for example, during GDT in human patients, the objectives of fluid resuscitation must be established based on the patient's needs. The objectives (*endpoints*) are different and depend on the patient's condition before hypovolemia set in (e.g., presence of renal or heart failure) and the ongoing pathological process (e.g., sepsis or severe dehydration), as indicated in Tables 3.6 and 3.7. Generally, the minimum effective fluid volume to achieve the targeted goal should be used, to avoid fluid accumulation in the various compartments in the postresuscitation phase.

Patients at highest risk of developing edema from aggressive fluid therapy are those with congestive heart failure, renal failure, pulmonary edema, and cerebral edema. In cats, hypothermia and peripheral vasoconstriction can promote the onset of edema, so it is important in this species to restore body temperature with active systems, such as devices that use hot air. The use of warm surfaces in contact with the patient's skin can cause plasmatic exemia, responsible for compartmentalized hypovolemia due to vasodilation in the contact area, which compromises an already impaired circulation.

Until the body temperature is restored to about 37 °C, small volume fluid resuscitation with minimum objectives is preferable, using balanced crystalloids in boluses of 5–15 mL over 20 minutes. Particular attention should also be paid to patients with a primary or secondary coagulopathy. The coagulation disorder of such patients may indeed be aggravated as a result of hemodilution or due to the interference of colloids with coagulation (see below); in addition, in patients with unstable clots (e.g., with traumatic bleeding), a sudden increase in systemic and capillary blood pressure can break down clots and aggravate bleeding.

In the absence of lesions that may alter the state of consciousness (e.g., head trauma), it should not be forgotten that the level of consciousness is a very useful parameter to evaluate the effectiveness of fluid therapy in restoring perfusion and brain oxygenation. Indeed, the recovery of consciousness or of a normal posture (e.g., patient standing up or lying in sternal recumbency) becomes clinically observable when a patient responds to fluid therapy, oxygenation, and the use of positive inotropic agents or vasoactive amines. Therefore, the state of consciousness can also be considered a monitoring parameter to evaluate the effectiveness of fluid resuscitation.

Chapter 3 ◆ Fluids: when and how to administer them

Fluid resuscitation with crystalloids

Fluid resuscitation with crystalloids is performed by administering IV boluses of 20–30 mL/kg over 15–20 minutes. Perfusion parameters are checked every 15–20 minutes; once they have been restored, fluid resuscitation is interrupted and daily fluid therapy is initiated. Generally, up to 3 IV 20 mL/kg boluses are administered in cats, and up to 4 IV 20 mL/kg boluses in dogs. When administering the penultimate bolus (the third in dogs and the second in cats), it is recommended to check for the presence of any vasodilation that might affect fluid therapy. It should be remembered that rapid administration of large volumes of crystalloids can cause glycocalyx damage (shedding) [24,25]. In addition, large volumes of crystalloids, especially when administered very quickly, can worsen the condition of patients with vasodilation (especially if renal failure is also present) and cause, for example, pulmonary and cerebral edema as well as generalized edema.

Fluid resuscitation with colloids

Colloids (Table 3.8) for fluid resuscitation should be administered IV; the usual shock dose in dogs is 10–20 mL/kg over 15–20 minutes. In cats they should be administered much more slowly, 5 mL/kg IV over 15–20 minutes: larger volumes and a faster administration may be responsible for neurological signs such as skeletal muscle tremor or CNS excitation. In a recent experimental study [26] conducted in pigs in which blood was collected until their baseline stroke volume index (SVI) dropped by 50% (about 500 mL of blood), 15 animals were administered a crystalloid solution (Ringer's lactate), while another 15 were administered a colloid solution (tetrastarch). All the animals underwent invasive and noninvasive monitoring of the following parameters: PPV, SVV, CI, MAP, $ScvO_2$, lactate, pH, and bicarbonate; laser Doppler flowmetry was used to assess blood flow in the microvascular system. To assess glycocalyx integrity, blood concentrations of syndecan-1 and glypican were quantified and showed that the glycocalyx was not damaged by the bleeding. The pigs were then provided fluid resuscitation with two types of fluids: for crystalloids it was necessary to administer about three times the lost volume (average of 1390 mL of Ringer's lactate solution, with a ratio of 3.03), while for colloids it was necessary to administer approximately the lost volume (average of 425 mL, with a ratio of 0.92). The study showed that, during acute bleeding (e.g., during surgery and trauma), the volume needed to restore the lost blood follows the Starling principle (crystalloids 3:1 and colloids 1:1), the glycocalyx remains intact, and colloids achieve hemodynamic stability more quickly. However, it should be remembered that in severely traumatized patients or those undergoing surgery with tissue damage, and in all cases in which glycocalyx damage may occur (sepsis, septic shock, hyperglycemia, systemic inflammation, and circulatory overload), the dynamics of the two types of fluids may change and the Starling principle of fluid exchange in the three compartments may no longer be valid (see Chapter 1).

Chapter 3 ◆ Fluids: when and how to administer them

Table 3.8 Composition of colloids

Solution	pH	Na+	Cl-	K+	Ca2+	Mg+	Osmolarity (mOsm/L)	Duration (hours)	BLOW	SID
Plasma	7.4	145	105	5	5	3	300	24	20	24
5% Albumin	7.4	130–160	130–160	0	0	0	310	24	20	0
6% Tetrastarch	5.7–6.5	154	154	0	0	0	308	4–6	25	33
6% Hetastarch	5.5	154	154	0	0	0	310	24	32	33
Dextran 70	5.1–5.7	154	154	0	0	0	310	24	59	0
Dextran 40	3.5–7.0	154	154	0	0	0	255	12	40	0
Gelatin	7.2–7.3	145	145	5.1	6.26	0	310	2–4	35	0
Succinyl-gelatin	7.4	154	125	0.4	0.4	0	279	2–4	35	0
3% NaCl	5.5	513	513	0	0	0	1025	2–4	0	0
7.5% NaCl	5.5	1283	1283	0	0	0	2567	2–4	0	0
18% Mannitol	4.5–7.0	0	0	0	0	0	988	2–4	0	0
HBOC	7.8	150	118	4	1.4	0	300	24	37	nd

Nd, not determined.

Chapter 3 ◆ Fluids: when and how to administer them

The adverse effects of fluid resuscitation with colloids are allergic reactions (25% especially with human albumin solution [25–30]) and coagulopathies, not due to hemodilution, which can also be caused by crystalloids, but to a specific antithrombotic action that hinders the polymerization of fibrin. The magnitude of this effect in the different colloids is, in descending order: dextran > hetastarch > pentastarch > tetrastarch > gelatin > albumin. In humans, the main reactions are related to, in descending order of frequency, gelatin (0.35%), dextran (0.27%), albumin (0.10%), and hydroxyethyl starches (0.06%). Severe reactions were recorded in sensitive patients in 20% of cases [31].

ROSE model (Resuscitation, Optimization, Stabilization, Evacuation)

Fluid therapy is usually used as a first treatment in critically and traumatized or hypovolemic patients. In the patients who respond to fluid therapy, i.e., those in the ascending part of the Starling curve (Figure 3.8), the increase in the venous compartment promotes an increase in the cardiac output and therefore in the hemodynamic parameters related to it (e.g., cardiac output and variation in ventricular ejection fraction). In practice, in human medicine it has been observed that only 50% of hemodynamically unstable patients are fluid responsive [30]. Aggressive fluid therapy without close hemodynamic monitoring (see Chapter 1) may be responsible for tissue edema and an obstacle to healing.

To optimize fluid therapy in critically ill or septic patients, the following subcategories have been proposed:
- Fluid resuscitation: aims to restore fluid losses with crystalloids or colloids; balanced crystalloid solutions are usually used.
- Daily fluid therapy with balanced isotonic solutions (see the Isotonic solutions section) that are in accordance with the patient's needs, in terms of volume of fluids and solution composition. In humans, a 10% increase in body weight is associated with a more unfavorable prognosis.
- Replacement fluid therapy: this corresponds to the fluids prepared based on the electrolytes and volume lost by the patient, and administered to replace losses (dehydration).
- Generalized increase in vascular permeability: it usually develops about 3 days after shock, during which vascular damage occurs due to cytokines and other proinflammatory molecules. At this stage, it is dangerous to perform aggressive fluid therapy as the risk of tissue edema is very high. At this stage it is advisable to switch to maintenance fluid therapy or, even better, to stop fluid therapy or maintain a zero fluid balance. The administration of fluids, at this stage, could fill

Chapter 3 ◆ Fluids: when and how to administer them

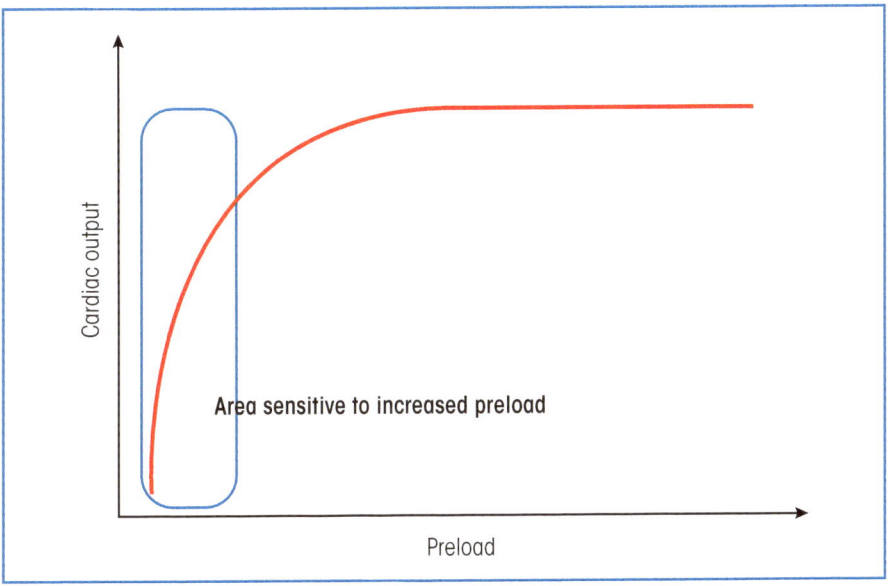

Figure 3.8 Variation of cardiac output by preload (Frank–Starling law).

the venous compartment only and increase its pressure without increasing the cardiac output-
- Fluid bolus: in humans, fluid boluses of 3–4 mL/kg over 10–15 minutes have been used. In veterinary medicine, before administering a fluid bolus of 20 mL/kg, a mini-fluid bolus of isotonic crystalloid solution may be administered at a dose of 3–5 mL/kg over 1 minute to check if the patient is fluid responsive. If the patient does not respond to both boluses (mini-fluid bolus and fluid bolus) it is likely non-fluid-responsive, due to damage to the vascular wall and glycocalyx, severe vasodilatation (e.g., sepsis), or heart failure;
- Evacuation: it is the phase during which the patient must eliminate excess fluids. This can be achieved through normal renal function, with the administration of drugs (e.g., furosemide) and, in very severe cases, with renal replacement therapy (RRT).

The acronym ROSE in reference to fluid therapy can be summarized as follows.
- Resuscitation (fluid resuscitation): it lasts a few minutes and corresponds to the phase during which fluids are administered quickly to restore the effective circulating volume in a hypovolemic patient (for example, with severe dehydration). Close hemodynamic monitoring is necessary at this stage.

Chapter 3 ◆ Fluids: when and how to administer them

- Optimization: in this phase, which lasts a few hours, the patient is always critical and hemodynamic monitoring must be performed, but the fluids are no longer administered through boluses and may be interrupted or infused at the maintenance rate. Tissue perfusion should be maintained.
- Stabilization: it follows the optimization phase, with an evolution over the next few days; in this phase a zero-fluid balance must be targeted and no accumulation of fluids must occur. During this phase, fluids are administered for maintenance and possibly to replace ongoing losses. In dogs and cats, an empirical but effective method to check for any fluid accumulation is to weigh the patient twice a day; better monitoring is achieved if this is combined with daily control of electrolytes, total proteins and hematocrit.
- Evacuation: this phase lasts from days to weeks. Typically, in our patients, it lasts only a few days (2–3 days) but it depends on the circulatory overload that may have occurred in the three previous phases. At this stage, fluid leakage from the vascular wall may occur. This means that the pathological process is still ongoing, and the patient may experience peripheral edema (pitting edema) or pulmonary edema (which manifests with tachypnea, hypoxia, and pulmonary congestion or edema, which can also be seen with a simple chest X-ray or TFAST). The patient may need supportive therapy to avoid fluid accumulation. In this phase, spontaneous fluid intake by the patient is encouraged (Box 3.6).

Crystalloids

Crystalloids are aqueous solutions containing small solutes that can crystallize and freely cross the vascular wall and interstitial compartment. As they move from the intravascular to the extravascular space (see Chapter 1), these solutes can cause a movement of water due to the concentration gradient. For this reason, most of these solutions contain large amounts of sodium, which not only contribute to ensure a similar osmolality to that of blood but also allow a larger volume of the water administered to remain inside the body and for a longer period than with water only. In fact, the administration of water only would cause the blood's osmotic pressure to drop and red blood cells to swell and eventually burst; in addition, such a solution administered in large amounts would cause tissue edema. In crystalloid solutions, one or more solutes are dissolved until an osmolality of about 300 mOsm/L is reached. Solutes are not metabolized by the patient, so their plasma concentration depends on their absorption and elimination. The chloride content of some solutions (e.g., balanced solutions) is significantly lower (about 40 mEq/L) than that of sodium; because chloride has a negative charge, negative charges are replaced by other molecules such as lactate, acetate, bicarbonate, or gluconate.

Chapter 3 ◆ Fluids: when and how to administer them

Box 3.6	Fluid therapy: ROSE acronym

- **R**esuscitation: fluid resuscitation and hemodynamic monitoring; lasts a few minutes.
- **O**ptimization: maintenance of effective circulation, hemodynamic monitoring; lasts a few hours.
- **S**tabilization: maintenance fluid therapy; lasts a few days. Weigh twice a day, check at least the hematocrit, total proteins, acid–base and electrolyte balance daily.
- **E**vacuation: it is done through the kidneys, but in the presence of vascular damage, leakage of fluids from the vascular wall may occur with subsequent edema (pulmonary, cerebral or peripheral); lasts a few days.

The famous pediatrician Alexis Hartmann added lactate (1930) to the balanced solution made by Sydney Ringer (1880) to treat metabolic acidosis in children, which is why the solution takes its name from him. In human medicine there is still some debate over whether it is appropriate to avoid infusing solutions with a high chloride concentration (e.g., saline solution) in critically ill patients during fluid resuscitation or when large volumes of fluids are infused to reduce mortality or hospitalization. The solutes, as they are not able to cross the cell membrane, remain in the extracellular fluid (ECF), where they normalize the osmolality of the intravascular and interstitial compartments. If the intracellular fluid (ICF) were to undergo an increase in osmolality, as occurs in severe forms of ICF dehydration (so-called cellular dehydration), water from the ECF would follow the concentration gradient and enter the cell and restore its osmolality and hydration.

Crystalloids are mainly used to restore the ECF, but thanks to their redistribution they can also be used to restore the ICF. The movement of water by osmotic gradient takes seconds, while the redistribution of electrolytes between the ICF and ECF spaces—which depends on the activity of the sodium–potassium pump and thus requires energy (produced in the mitochondria in the form of ATP) and oxygen—takes minutes to hours. The distribution of fluids can be represented using the two-volume model [23,24], which states that when the vc (the expanded central body fluid space) is close to the Vc (same body fluid space at baseline), the increase in volume is close to zero; when this happens, the total clearance of water is close to Clo (sum of all fluid losses) (Figure 3.9). This means that the distribution between the Vc and the Vt (interstitial fluid volume), or Jv, depends on the osmotic gradients multiplied by clearance, while elimination takes place from the Vc and is proportional to plasma dilution multiplied by the Cl (losses caused by fluid therapy). When the elimination of the administered fluid is complete, redistribution occurs, that is, fluid

Chapter 3 ◆ Fluids: when and how to administer them

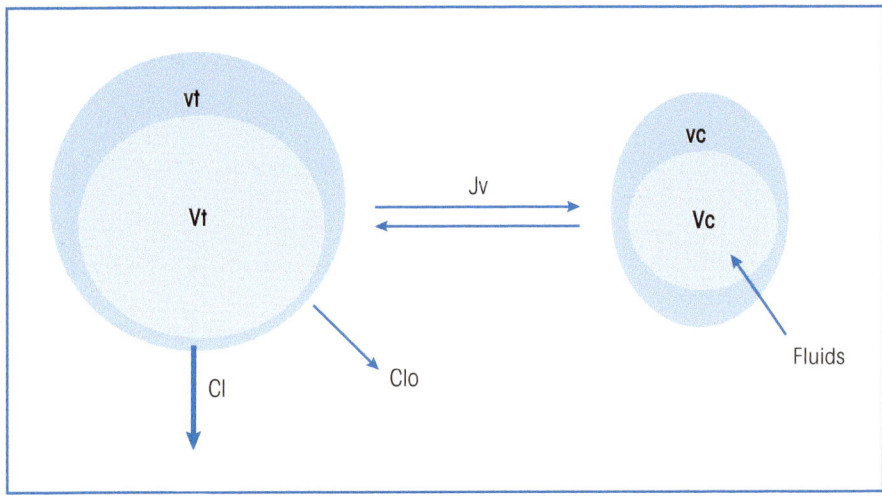

Figure 3.9 Fluid kinetics, two-volume model: when fluid administration causes an expansion of vascular volume (Vc), an increase in Cl occurs; when vc is close to Vc, Cl is close to Clo (see text). Cl, losses resulting from fluid therapy; Clo, insensitive leaks; Jv, transvascular flow; Vc, intravascular space; vc, expanded intravascular space; Vt, interstitial fluid volume; vt, Vt expanded with fluids.

passes from Vt to Vc [23]. In humans, the distribution of crystalloids stops during episodes of acute hypotension (e.g, during anesthesia), and their redistribution is also hindered by rapid infusions and probably by large volumes; their elimination is reduced by hypotension [23].

Intravenously infused crystalloids have a short half-life; in humans, when the vascular wall is intact (healthy patients), it is about 60 minutes for Ringer's lactate and 130 minutes for saline solution. Their distribution from plasma to the interstitial space occurs over about 20–30 minutes (Box 3.7). Of course, in patients with vascular and glycocalyx damage, their distribution will be altered and they may remain in the vascular compartment for a shorter period of time, as occurs for example in patients with sepsis or systemic inflammation.

Crystalloids are considered the first choice of fluids to restore the ECF volume and are also used for fluid resuscitation, given that the revision of Starling's principle has shown that, at low capillary pressures (<20 mmHg), crystalloids remain in the circulation like colloids.

Crystalloids can be administered intravenously or subcutaneously. The latter route of administration is only used when crystalloids cannot be administered intravenously due to the impossibility of hospitalizing the patient for 24 hours. In such special cases, the largest possible volume is administered intravenously, and the remainder (usually

Chapter 3 ◆ Fluids: when and how to administer them

Box 3.7	Crystalloids

- Crystalloids: aqueous solutions that contain small solutes, e.g., 0.9% NaCl, Ringer, 5% glucose
- Isotonic saline solution: crystalloid solution with a plasma-like osmotic pressure
- "**Balanced**" isotonic solutions: solutions with a concentration of electrolytes similar to that of plasma (e.g., Ringer's lactate); used in maintenance fluid therapy but also in fluid resuscitation
- "**Unbalanced**" solutions: solutions with a concentration of electrolytes different to that to plasma (e.g., 0.9% NaCl, 5% glucose); mainly used in maintenance fluid therapy
- Crystalloids are distributed in the three compartments (intravascular, interstitial and intracellular) in about 30 minutes
- Daily fluid dose: 1–2 mL/kg/day. Fluid resuscitation dose: maximum of 4 boluses 20 mL/kg over 15–20 min IV in dogs; in cats, maximum of 3 boluses

the night dose) is administered subcutaneously. When using this route, it is essential not to administer hypertonic solutions, because they have a tissue-damaging action; up to 600–700 mOsm/L can be administered intravenously. Subcutaneous administration is not effective in quickly correcting electrolyte imbalances because fluids must be reabsorbed from the interstitial space, where electrolytes can be retained and, if they are present in high concentrations, cause inflammation. The addition of electrolytes to balanced crystalloid solutions (e.g., potassium chloride) administered subcutaneously may be responsible for cutaneous and subcutaneous inflammation, ulcers, and necrosis with loss of skin barrier integrity. The maximum recommended dose to be administered subcutaneously is approximately 1–1.5% of the body weight.

Crystalloids are also classified as isotonic, hypotonic, or hypertonic, based on their osmolality with respect to that of plasma (see Table 3.1). Isotonic crystalloids are mainly used as maintenance fluids, while hypotonic crystalloids are used when it is necessary to administer fluids that are retained within the circulatory system for the shortest possible time (e.g., half strength in congestive heart failure). Another example of a hypotonic solution is *5% glucose*. The osmolality of this solution is about 50 mEq/L lower than that of plasma and it is mainly used to administer water, glucose, and a modest caloric intake (0.17 kcal/mL). It does not contain any electrolytes; therefore, it is not used as a maintenance fluid and has an acidic pH (about 5.0). It is often used to maintain blood sugar levels and is added to other crystalloids to reduce their osmolality. When the objective is to administer water only, the glucose contained in the solution is transformed very quickly into CO_2 and water.

Chapter 3 ◆ Fluids: when and how to administer them

Isotonic solutions

Isotonic saline solutions are the most commonly used solutions. Saline, when prepared with *0.9% NaCl*, has a plasma-like osmolality, but a higher concentration of sodium and especially of chloride than plasma (about 50 mEq/L more than plasma). The administration of saline can cause metabolic acidosis, because chloride is negatively charged and therefore causes an increase in protons (H^+), as saline does not contain bicarbonate or other buffer molecules of acidic chemical species.

Saline solution is used to correct hypochloremic metabolic alkalosis, as a maintenance fluid, to correct hyponatremia (caused, for example, by vomiting and polyuria), and for fluid resuscitation. It is the most commonly used solution in human medicine and is also used in hospitalized patients as a vehicle for the administration of drugs; it can be responsible for hypernatremia or hyperchloremia. There is no data available on its frequency of administration in veterinary medicine. Due to its high sodium concentration, it remains longer in the circulation (about 10%) than other balanced solutions (e.g., Ringer's lactate). Because it does not contain calcium, it is also used to administer drugs that are not compatible with other solutions, such as bicarbonate, whole blood, or blood products that contain anticoagulants that chelate calcium.

Ringer's solutions are named after the physiologist who first prepared them after observing, in his studies on animal models, that the administration of a solution containing more electrolytes, such as sodium, potassium, calcium, and chloride, was able to preserve protoplasmic activities, unlike simple water. Ringer's solutions contain about 30 mEq/L of buffer, in the form of acetate or lactate. Both types provide a very low caloric intake (about 5 kcal/L). Acetate is metabolized more quickly than lactate and in more tissues (e.g., liver and muscles). In addition, this process requires half the oxygen needed to metabolize lactate.

During hepatic failure, acetate is transformed in the kidney into ketone bodies, which are useful as a source of energy [31]. Rapid administration of Ringer's acetate may be responsible for a reduction in SVR. During shock in dogs, the metabolism of acetate is preserved while that of lactate is reduced [32]. In humans, acetate increases the bicarbonate concentration after only 15 minutes and has a greater alkalizing activity than lactate [33]. Because acetate is not converted into glucose like lactate, it does not cause hyperglycemia. This phenomenon becomes especially important when administering fluids in diabetic patients. Ringer's solutions cannot be used when administering substances that are incompatible with calcium, such as certain drugs, blood products, or whole blood (incompatible with the sodium citrate contained in the anticoagulant). Their elimination is very rapid and is slowed down during hypotension and general anesthesia (in humans, under normal conditions, about 70% is eliminated in 2 hours). Ringer's solutions are used in fluid resuscitation and in daily fluid therapy when the patient's electrolyte and acid–base status is unknown, so as to reduce the risk of electrolyte and acid–base imbalances, given that the composition of these solutions is close to that of plasma.

Plasma-Lyte is another isotonic solution of balanced electrolytes used predominantly to correct metabolic acidosis, as it contains about 50 bicarbonate precursors. Its concentration in sodium and chloride is close to that of plasma and it does not contain calcium but magnesium, which can be useful to correct refractory hypokalemia. Hypokalemia is very frequent in critically ill patients, especially those with ECF imbalances (e.g., with vomiting and diarrhea). Gluconate has a lower alkalizing effect than acetate. Since it does not contain calcium, this solution can also be used when administering substances that are incompatible with calcium, such as certain drugs, blood products or whole blood. This isotonic solution is preferred in the therapy of renal failure, as it contains more buffers to treat metabolic acidosis and a number of ions more similar to that of plasma than other isotonic solutions. It is also used to treat patients in shock and when the patient's electrolyte and acid–base status is unknown.

Hypertonic solutions

Hypertonic solutions are used when the objective is to expand the circulating volume. A sudden increase (a few seconds or minutes) in blood osmolality thanks to the created osmotic gradient can lead to an expansion of the circulating volume proportional to its concentration. A typical hypertonic solution is *7.5% NaCl*, because it can draw water into the intravascular compartment by osmotic gradient in a few seconds and therefore expands the plasma volume very quickly. It is also used in patients with cerebral edema, to reduce its extent, and is administered at a dose of 2–5 mL/kg IV. Due to its high osmolality, 7.5% NaCl should only be administered intravenously. Before administration it should be checked that the patient is not severely hyponatremic, because too rapid an increase in serum sodium can cause severe neurological lesions (e.g., pontine myelinolysis), even 2–3 days after administration. To check if the administration of this fluid has caused an electrolyte disorder it is necessary to wait at least 30 minutes, so that the solution can be redistributed. Its use is also advised against in cases of hypernatremia and severe dehydration: its rapid administration can cause hypertension and bradycardia.

Another frequently used hypertonic solution is *18% mannitol*. It draws water from the extravascular space through the osmotic gradient produced by its high osmolality (about 988 mOsm/L). It is therefore administered exclusively intravenously and is irritant to the vascular walls. Mannitol should only be administered in hemodynamically stable patients and is used in cases of head trauma as it can reduce cerebral edema. In such cases, it is administered at a dose of 500 mg/kg IV over 15–20 minutes. Typically, 3–4 boluses are administered at an interval of 2–6 hours, depending on the severity of the edema and the response to therapy. The diuretic effect after administration in boluses occurs over approximately 20 minutes. In patients at risk of hypervolemia, such as those with congestive heart failure or kidney failure, hemodynamic parameters should be closely monitored. In these patients, the administration of mannitol may cause an increase in the respiratory rate due to pulmonary congestion or pulmonary edema. Mannitol, thanks to its hypertonicity, causes osmotic diuresis by drawing water into the nephron, reduces blood viscosity, improves blood flow in the kidneys and capillaries, and reduces edema of the epithelial tubular cells and obstruction of the tubular lumen caused by casts and cell debris; in addition, it eliminates free radicals.

Colloids

Colloids are aqueous solutions that contain macromolecules of such size that they are not able to cross the vascular wall under normal conditions (intact vascular wall) and therefore increase the oncotic pressure in the intravascular compartment. The degradation of these macromolecules affects the permanence of the colloid in the intravascular compartment. The size, molecular weight, and chemical structure of these molecules affect the oncotic pressure and dynamics of the fluids. The shorter the degradation time of the macromolecules, the shorter the duration of their effect. Because they do not generate a sufficient osmotic pressure, they must be combined with some electrolytes to maintain an osmotic pressure that will not cause intravascular hemolysis. For this reason, colloid solutions are prepared with normal saline, Ringer's lactate or other isotonic saline solutions. Their kinetics are one-compartment, that is, the administered fluid does not distribute through the various compartments but is used to expand the intravascular volume. In this sense, colloids are more effective and rapid than crystalloids.

They are also used to restore the circulating volume in case of hemorrhage with a blood loss equal to or greater than 10–15% of the circulating volume. Recently, their use has been questioned in human medicine, as it has been reported that hydroxyethyl starches can increase the risk of renal failure and mortality. Therefore, their use is not recommended in patients with sepsis, septic shock, kidney failure, or head trauma, or in case of organ donation [34,35]. Colloids can be divided into synthetic and natural colloids (Box 3.8).

Chapter 3 ◆ Fluids: when and how to administer them

Box 3.8	Colloids

- Colloids: aqueous solutions that contain large solutes, from 30 kDa to 450 kDa
- Synthetic colloids: dextran, hydroxyethyl starches
- Natural colloids: plasma, canine albumin, human albumin, gelatin, HBOC (hemoglobin-based oxygen-carrying solution)
- Daily dose: 10–20 mL/kg/day. Resuscitation dose: in dogs, they can be administered in a single bolus; in cats, in boluses of 5 mL/kg IV over 15–20 min. In both species the doses can be administered as a CRI of 2 mL/kg/hour.

Synthetic colloids

The most commonly used synthetic colloids are dextran-70 and hydroxyethyl starches, while natural colloids are gelatin, species-specific plasma, and canine and human albumin. The major limitations to their use are allergic reactions and their high cost compared to crystalloids. The maximum recommended dose is 20 mL/kg/day IV; colloids cannot be administered subcutaneously. Higher doses may be responsible for coagulopathies and circulatory overload, as well as for an increased risk of hypersensitivity reactions [37]. The recommended maintenance rate is 2 mL/kg/hour IV. This type of administration is preferred when there is chronic or continuous plasma protein leakage (e.g., protein-losing enteropathy, gastrointestinal form of parvovirus disease).

Dextran solutions are aqueous solutions containing long-chain glucose molecules (polysaccharides) with a high molecular weight, derived from the fermentation of glucose by specific bacteria (*Leuconostoc mesenteroides* or lactobacilli). Like other colloids, polysaccharides also have a low osmolality and need to be dissolved in crystalloids such as normal saline, Ringer's solution or hypertonic saline (rescue solution). Dextran solutions can contain polysaccharides with a high average molecular weight, such as dextran-70 (70 kDa), or with a lower molecular weight, such as dextran-40 (40 kDa). The most commonly used dextran solution is 6% dextran-70, since it expands the circulating volume by a volume equal to that infused, while dextran-40 can cause tubular obstruction or renal failure, especially in dehydrated patients. The effect of dextran-70 is long-lasting (about 24 hours) and it has a positive rheological activity that makes the surface of cells (blood cells, platelets and white blood cells) less adhesive, thus reducing blood viscosity and improving capillary blood flow; however, it can prolong clotting times. For these reasons, dextran solutions should be used with caution and under close monitoring during surgery, in patients with bleeding, or in those with a coagulation disorder (e.g., disseminated intravascular coagu-

Chapter 3 ◆ Fluids: when and how to administer them

lation). Thanks to the above mentioned properties, dextran can be used to expand the circulating volume and prevent the formation of thrombi. Dextran solutions are administered at a dose of 10–20 mL/kg/day. The rescue solution should be administered as a bolus at a dose of 2–4 mL/kg IV (in dogs). Like other colloids, in the cat they should be administered much more slowly: 5 mL/ kg IV over 15–20 minutes.

Hydroxyethyl starches (HES) are amylopectins derived from corn or wheat, dissolved in isotonic crystalloids (e.g., saline or Ringer's solution). HES are also dissolved in hypertonic solutions such as dextran-70 and hypertonic saline solution. HES are used in fluid resuscitation to expand the circulating volume by a greater volume than that infused. Amylopectins are hydroxylated because they would otherwise be degraded very quickly by plasma amylases. HES are a mixture of smaller molecules (50–70 kDa), which are quickly excreted through the kidneys, and larger molecules than average, which are degraded by amylases and partly phagocytosed by the reticuloendothelial system, so that it is possible in humans to detect them in the liver and spleen for years [35,36]. The number and position of hydroxylations (OH groups) present in amylopectin molecules modify their biological behavior. Molecular weight and concentration (6–10%) are also responsible for the activity of the solution; therefore, to know the blood volume expansion capacity and duration of effect of a HES, its molecular weight, the C2/C6 ratio, and the degree of substitution should be identified. The degree of substitution varies from 0.4 to 0.8: the higher the degree of substitution, the greater the resistance of the HES to degradation by amylases, and therefore the longer its persistence in the vascular bed. Solutions with a low degree of substitution (0.4) are generally preferred. The C_2/C_6 ratio, which indicates the position of the OH groups, affects the half-life and thus the persistence of the HES in blood. Values ≥8 are considered high, while values of 4–5 are preferred. The molecular weight can be high, as in hetastarch, which has a molecular weight of about 450 kDa and thus is the HES with the greatest duration of effect (about 24 hours). Pentastarch has an intermediate molecular weight of 260 kDa, while tetrastarch has the lowest molecular weight (130 kDa) and consequently a shorter duration of effect, about 2–4 hours. Sixty percent of tetrastarch molecules can be found in the urine for 72 hours.

The duration of effect of HES may be prolonged in states of hypotension, and it is greater after a hemorrhage. The higher the molecular weight, the greater the risk of hypersensitivity reactions and coagulopathies. In humans, the perception of subcutaneous tingling has been described; it can last for months and, in severe cases, even up to 2 years. This has not been reported in animals.

Solutions containing molecules weighing 50 kDa or less have a very short shelf-life of about 2–4 hours. Tetrastarch is preferred over the other two types of HES, because its duration usually allows stabilization of critical patients. The most commonly used solutions have a molecular weight of 130 kDa, a degree of substitution of 0.4, and a $C_2/$

Chapter 3 ◆ Fluids: when and how to administer them

C_6 ratio of 9:1 (Voluven®), or a molecular weight of 130 kDa, a degree of substitution of 0.62, and a C_2/C_6 ratio of 6:1 (Venofundin®).

In humans, the main indication for the administration of HES is the expansion of the circulating volume in patients suffering from bleeding, while its use in intensive care is not recommended. The dose used in dogs and cats is 10–20 mL/kg/day IV; in cats they should be administered much more slowly (5 mL/kg IV over 15–20 minutes).

Natural colloids

Albumin is the plasma protein with the highest concentration; it has a molecular weight of about 70 kDa and can generate 3/4 of the oncotic blood pressure. Its particular symmetrical quaternary structure and its negative charge (-19) allow it to bind to ions, lipids, metals, hormones and drugs. It transports and binds to various biologically active molecules, it is anti-inflammatory and antioxidant, it stabilizes the endothelium, it is present in the glycocalyx, it has antiplatelet activity, and it contributes to the acid–base balance. The synthesis of albumin occurs mainly in the liver and is induced by osmoreceptors located in the interstitial space of the liver. Its reduction is a marker of hepatic function deficiency. Its production is reduced if its concentration is high; the hepatic capillaries, as they are fenestrated, allow osmoreceptors to perceive increased levels of albumin. For this reason, the intravenous administration of albumin at high concentrations (e.g., 20%) can cause an inhibition of its synthesis. Decreased blood albumin levels can be caused by peritonitis, pleurisy, liver disease, kidney failure, protein-losing enteropathy, pericardiectomy, and neoplasms. The biological activity of some drugs and calcium (see Chapter 4) depends on its concentration; the patient's plasma albumin concentration should therefore be evaluated before administering it. The drugs most affected by serum albumin concentration are many antibiotics, diazepam, midazolam, thiopental, nonsteroidal anti-inflammatory drugs, digoxin, and warfarin.

In addition to expanding the circulating volume, albumin helps to reduce transvascular flow when the capillary hydrostatic pressure increases, improves the microcirculation by modifying the laminar blood flow, and contributes to increasing blood pressure by expanding the circulating volume and to the removal of many reactive chemical species, such as superoxides, some cations, anions, and many inflammatory molecules, especially those with a positive charge. The polynitroxylated albumin that forms in the circulation, thereby increasing the redox potential, protects cells from reperfusion injury and inhibits xanthine oxidase, which is responsible for cell death.

For the reasons mentioned above, the administration of human albumin (HSA, human serum albumin) constitutes a therapeutic option to be considered during septic shock (not for fluid resuscitation, see below). Its higher concentration in the

Chapter 3 ◆ Fluids: when and how to administer them

intravascular compartment (4 g/dL) than in the extravascular compartment (1.4 g/dL) creates an essential osmotic gradient for the passage of fluids from the intravascular to the extravascular space (see Chapter 1). The passage of albumin from the intravascular to the extravascular compartment is called TER (transcapillary escape rate). TER is conditioned by the integrity of the vascular wall, the glycocalyx, the serum albumin concentration and subglycocalyx space, the volume of water in plasma and the electrical charges present on the two sides of the vessel wall. The pathological processes that most frequently alter the TER are sepsis, septic shock, systemic inflammation, severe trauma, pneumonia, hyperosmolar syndrome, heat stroke, ischemic diseases, burns, animal poisons, autoimmune diseases, and systemic neoplasms.

The leakage of albumin from the vascular bed, which under normal conditions is about 5%, can reach 20% during sepsis due to glycocalyx damage. To normalize the TER rapidly, albumin can be administered slowly by an intravenous constant rate infusion (CRI). On the market there are HSA preparations at 3.5%, 5%, 20%, 25%. Canine albumin is also available in some countries. HSA at 5% is iso-oncotic compared to blood (308 mOsm/L), while 25% HSA is hyperoncotic (1500 mOsm/L). Five percent HSA can expand the circulating volume in 30–60 minutes, by a volume close to the infused one. Its effect lasts about 24 hours and it is used when albumin is less than 2 g/dL or in cases of severe and continuous losses.

It should be remembered that hypoalbuminemia is the sign of a disease and not a disease in itself, so it is recommended to first treat the pathological process that caused it, and only when losses are continuous and may cause complications should albumin be administered. The volume to be administered is 10–20 mL/kg/day IV. It should be diluted until a 5% solution is obtained and administered as a CRI at a rate of 2 mL/kg/hour IV, which corresponds to a 5- to 10-hour infusion, during which the serum albumin concentration is normalized and clinical hemodynamic benefits can be observed. The above dose can be repeated daily and for several days, as needed by the patient. In the author's experience, 5% HSA has been administered daily for up to 11 consecutive days in dogs. At these doses and rate, and even with repeated daily administrations in the same patient (dog or cat), the author has never observed any hypersensitivity reactions over the course of 30 years of administration in dogs and cats [38]. The author administers 20% HSA by diluting it to 5% in saline or Ringer's solution depending on the patient's needs (acid–base and electrolyte status), according to the protocol indicated above [36]. HSA should not be administered at high concentrations and during fluid resuscitation due to the high risk of type I hypersensitivity reactions (e.g., anaphylactic shock), especially when administered at 25%.

Adverse effects, in addition to possible hypersensitivity reactions, are comparable to those of other colloids: hemodilution, reduction in the concentration of coagulation factors, and circulatory overload. When administered, patients should be closely

Chapter 3 ◆ Fluids: when and how to administer them

monitored for type I hypersensitivity reactions, such as tremors, hyperthermia, facial and laryngeal edema, bronchospasm, hypotension, and anaphylactic shock. Rapid administration of albumin may impair its peripheral lymphatic reabsorption, so it is recommended to administer it slowly (2 mL/kg/hour). Studies in human medicine [39,40] have demonstrated a survival benefit in septic shock patients.

Albumin administration is therefore recommended in acute hypoalbuminemia, since in chronic forms (e.g., in cases of leishmaniasis), the presence of circulating globulins generally compensates for the deficient colloid osmotic pressure (COP). It is not recommended to administer human albumin during cardiopulmonary resuscitation and over 1 g/kg/day (20 mL/kg/day of 5% HAS), due to the increased risk of type I hypersensitivity reactions.

Species-specific plasma must belong to the same blood type as the receiving patient. For this reason, before administering it, it is good to test the recipient's blood type. Due to its high cost and scarce availability, it is mainly used to treat secondary coagulopathies (coagulation factor deficiency) and, to a lesser extent, to treat hypoproteinemia. Plasma, which contains numerous proteins, may be responsible for type I and type III hypersensitivity reactions. The first are the typical reactions that occur shortly after plasma administration (minutes or hours), causing tremors, hyperthermia, facial and laryngeal edema, bronchospasm, hypotension, and anaphylactic shock. Type III hypersensitivity reactions are characterized by the formation of antigen–antibody immunocomplexes that may result in vasculitis, glomerulonephritis, arthritis, vesicular or ulcerative dermatitis, and hemolytic anemia. These last reactions can occur after several days and for up to 3–4 weeks.

Fresh plasma, in order to preserve coagulation factors, must be separated from whole blood within 8 hours of its collection and stored at a temperature of 1–6 °C. Fresh plasma can be kept refrigerated for up to 6 weeks, after which it must be frozen at –18 °C. In addition to coagulation factors, plasma, whether fresh or fresh frozen, contains albumin, fibronectin, antitrypsin, and antithrombin III. Plasma frozen for more than 1 year and up to 5 years no longer contains effective coagulation factors, so it can only be used, after slow thawing, for the administration of plasma proteins. The dose for administration of coagulation factors or plasma proteins is 10–20 mL/kg/day IV.

Gelatin is a product obtained from the thermal chemical hydrolysis of bovine bone collagen. This was one of the first colloids to be made for medical purposes; in fact, its use dates to the First World War, when Bayliss made a solution containing 5% gelatin to treat patients in shock. Gelatin can have a reticular structure with urea bridges (e.g., Emagel® 3.5%), or be composed of succinyl-gelatin (Eufusin® 4%) or modified fluid gelatin (Gelplex® 3%). Succinyl-gelatin has higher negative charges, which give it a greater oncotic activity, and in humans it has a lower risk of anaphylaxis. In humans, gelatin interferes less with coagulation [41]. Because it has a very

Chapter 3 ◆ Fluids: when and how to administer them

low molecular weight (30 kDa), it is eliminated mainly through the kidneys and has a short duration of action of about 2 hours. This short duration of action can be a downside but also an advantage, since, if gelatin is used to quickly restore the circulating volume (fluid resuscitation), it will expand it to an extent comparable to HES, but for a shorter period of time and without interfering with the continuation of therapy. Gelatin is easily available and costs less than other colloids. It also interferes less with coagulation than HES. In humans, hypersensitivity reactions are greater with gelatin than with HES and dextran; no data about this is available in veterinary medicine. The daily dose is 10–20 mL/kg IV.

References

[1] National Research Council. *Water. Nutrient requirements of dogs and cats*. Washington, DC: National Academy Press; 2006. pp. 246–251.

[2] Hansen B, Vigani A. Maintenance fluid therapy isotonic versus hypotonic solutions. *Vet Clin Small Anim*. 2017;47:383–395.

[3] Cecconi M, Hofer C, Teboul JL et al. FENICE Investigators; ESICM Trial Group. Fluid challenges in intensive care: the FENICE study. A global inception cohort study. *Intensive Care Med*. 2015;41(9):1529–1537.

[4] McNab S, Duke T, South M et al. 140 mmol/L of sodium versus 77 mmol/L of sodium in maintenance intravenous fluid therapy for children in hospital (PIMS): a randomised controlled double-blind trial. *Lancet*. 2015;385:1190–1197.

[5] Van Regenmortel T, De Weerd T, Van Craenenbroeck E et al. Effect of isotonic versus hypotonic maintenance fluid therapy on urine output, fluid balance, and electrolyte homeostasis: a crossover study in fasting adult volunteers. *Br J Anaesth*. 2017 Jun;118(6):892–900.

[6] Hauptman JG, Richter MA, Wood SL et al. Effects of anesthesia, surgery, and intravenous administration of fluids on plasma antidiuretic hormone concentrations in healthy dogs. *Am J Vet Res*. 2000;61:1273–1276.

[7] Lamke LO, Nilsson GE, Reithner HL. Water loss by evaporation from abdominal cavity during surgery. *Acta Chir Scand*. 1977;143:279–284.

[8] Roe CF. Effect of bowel exposure on body temperature during surgical operation. *Am J Surg*. 1971;122.

[9] Myles P, Bellomo R, Corcoran T et al. Restrictive versus liberal fluid therapy in major abdominal surgery (RELIEF): rationale and design for a multicentre randomised trial. *BMJ Open*. 2017;7:e015358.

[10] Cabrales P, Martini J, Intaglietta M et al. Blood viscosity maintains microvascular conditions during normovolemic anemia independent of blood-oxygen carrying capacity. *Am J Physiol Heart Circ Physiol*. 2006;291(2):H581–590.

Chapter 3 ◆ Fluids: when and how to administer them

[11] Ospina-Tascon G, Neves AP, Occhipinti G. Effects of fluids on microvascular perfusion in patients with severe sepsis. *Intensive Care Med.* 2010 Jun;36(6):949–955.

[12] Grocott MP, Martin DS, Levett DZ, Arterial blood gases and oxygen content in climbers on Mount Everest. *N Engl J Med.* 2009 Jan 8;360(2):140–149.

[13] Garcia-Alvarez M, Marik P, Bellomo R. Sepsis-associated hyperlactatemia. *Crit Care.* 2014 Sep 9;18(5):503.

[14] Kalantari K, Chang JN, Ronco C et al. Assessment of intravascular volume status and volume responsiveness in critically ill patients. *Kidney International.* 2013;83:1017–1028.

[15] Shoemaker W, Appel PL, Kram HB. Prospective trial of supranormal values of survivors as therapeutics goals in high-risk surgical patients. *Chest.* 1988 Dec;94(6):1176–1186.

[16] Grocott MP, Dushianthan A, Hamilton MA et al. Optimisation Systematic Review Steering Group. Perioperative increase in global blood flow to explicit defined goals and outcomes after surgery: a Cochrane Systematic Review. *Br J Anaesth.* 2013 Oct;111(4):535–548.

[17] Pearse RM, Harrison DA, MacDonald N et al. The OPTIMISE Study Group. Effect of a perioperative, cardiac output-guided hemodynamic therapy algorithm on outcomes following major gastrointestinal surgery: a randomized clinical trial and systematic review. *JAMA.* 2014 Jun 4; 311(21):2181–2190.

[18] Perel P, Roberts I, Ker K. Colloids versus crystalloids for fluid resuscitation in critically ill patients. *Cochrane Database Syst Rev.* 2013 Feb 28;2:CD000567.

[19] Annane D, Siami S, Jaber S et al. Effects of fluid resuscitation with colloids vs crystalloids on mortality in critically ill patients presenting with hypovolemic shock: the CRISTAL randomized trial. JAMA. 2013 Nov 6;310(17):1809–1817.

[20] Adamik KN, Yozova ID, Regenscheit N. Controversies in the use of hydroxyethyl starch solutions in small animal emergency and critical care. *J Vet Emerg Crit Care.* 2015;25(1):20–47.

[21] Yozova ID, Howard J, Adamik KN. Retrospective evaluation of the effects of administration of tetrastarch (hydroxyethyl starch 130/0.4) on plasma creatinine concentration in dogs (2010-2013): 201 dogs. *J Vet Emerg Crit Care.* 2016 Jul;26(4):568–577.

[22] Hayes G, Benedicenti L, Mathews K. Retrospective cohort study on the incidence of acute kidney injury and death following hydroxyethyl starch (HES 10% 250/0.5/5:1) administration in dogs (2007-2010). *J Vet Emerg Crit Care.* 2016 Jan-Feb;26(1):35–40.

[23] Hahn RG. Volume kinetics for infusion fluids. *Anesthesiology.* 2010 Aug;113(2):470–481.

[24] Smart L, Boyd CJ et al. Large-Volume Crystalloid Fluid Is Associated with Increased Hyaluronan Shedding and Inflammation in a Canine Hemorrhagic Shock Model. *Inflammation.* 2018 Aug;41(4):1515–1523.

[25] Yiew X, Bateman SW, Hahn RG et al. Understanding Volume Kinetics: The Role of Pharmacokinetic Modeling and Analysis in Fluid Therapy. *Front Vet Sci.* 2020 Nov 20;7:587106.

Chapter 3 ◆ Fluids: when and how to administer them

[26] László I, Demeter G, Öveges N. Volume-replacement ratio for crystalloids and colloids during bleeding and resuscitation: an animal experiment. *Intensive Care Med Exp*. 2017 Dec;5:52.

[27] Martin L, Luther T, Alperin DC et al. Serum antibodies against human albumin in critically ill and healthy dogs. *J Am Vet Med Assoc*. 2008;232(7):1004–1009.

[28] Cohn L, Kerl M, Lenox CE et al. Response of healthy dogs to infusions of human serum albumin. *Am J Vet Res*. 2007;68(6):657–663.

[29] Laxenaire MC, Charpentier C, Feldman L. Anaphylactoid reactions to colloid plasma substitutes: incidence, risk factors, mechanisms. A French multicenter prospective study. *Ann Fr Anesth Reanim*. 1994;13(3):301–310.

[30] Marik PE, Monnet X, Teboul JL. Haemodynamic parameters to guide fluid therapy. *Ann Intensive Care*. 2011;1:1.

[31] Nakatani T. Overview of the effects of Ringer's acetate solution and a new concept: renal ketogenesis during hepatic inflow occlusion. *Methods Find Exp Clin Pharmacol*. 2001 Nov;23(9):519–528.

[32] Nakatani T. Utilization of exogenous acetate during canine hemorrhagic shock. *Scand J Clin Lab Invest*. 1979;39(7).

[33] Hamada T, Yamamoto M, Nakamaru K et al. The pharmacokinetics of D-lactate, L-lactate and acetate in humans. *Masui*. 1997 Feb;46(2):229–236.

[34] Reinhart K, Perner A, Sprung CL. Consensus statement of the ESICM task force on colloid volume therapy in critically ill patients. *Intensive Care Med*. 2012 Mar;38(3):368–383.

[35] Zarychanski R, Abou-Setta AM, Turgeon AF. Association of hydroxyethyl starch administration with mortality and acute kidney injury in critically ill patients requiring volume resuscitation: a systematic review and meta-analysis. *JAMA*. 2013 Feb 20;309(7):678–688.

[36] Sirtl C, Laubenthal H, Zumtobel V et al. Tissue deposits of hydroxyethyl starch (HES): dose-dependent and time-related. *Br J Anaesth*. 1999 Apr;82(4):510–515.

[37] Thompson WL, Fukushima T, Rutherford RB et al. Intravascular persistence, tissue storage, and excretion of hydroxyethyl starch. *Surg Gynecol Obstet*. 1970 Nov;131(5):965–972.

[38] Viganò F, Perissinotto L, Bosco V. Administration of 5% human serum albumin in critically ill small animal patients with hypoalbuminemia: 418 dogs and 170 cats (1994-2008). *J Vet Emerg Crit Care*. 2010;20(2):237–243.

[39] Caironi P, Tognoni G, Masson S. Albumin replacement in patients with severe sepsis or septic shock (ALBIOS). *N Engl J Med*. 2014; 370:1412–1421.

[40] Finfer S, Bellomo R, Boyce N. A comparison of albumin and saline for fluid resuscitation in the intensive care unit (SAFE). *N Engl J Med*. 2004 May 27;350(22):2247–2256.

[41] Haas T, Preinreich A, Oswald E. Effects of albumin 5% and artificial colloids on clot formation in small infants. *Anaesthesia*. 2007 Oct;62(10):1000–1007.

Clinical Case

Consequences of gastroenteritis

Prevalence				
Technical difficulty				

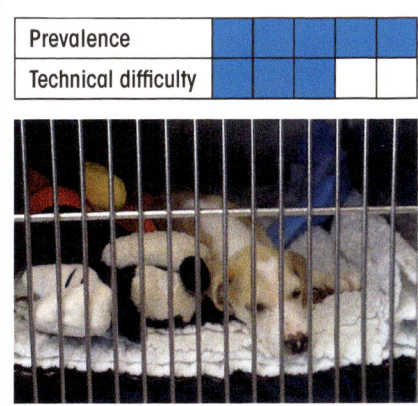

Signalment	
Name	Jack
Species	canine
Breed	mixed breed
Sex	intact male
Weight	12 kg
Age	6 months

History

The patient was taken for a medical examination because he had been showing anorexia for 3 days, with about five episodes of vomiting per day (described as gastric juice) and four episodes of diarrhea with blood. The owner explained that the dog refused to take food, even when offered by hand, and that he kept vomiting shortly after drinking. Abdominal pain and intestinal loop enlargement were detected on physical examination.

The initial examination revealed the following vital parameters:
- heart rate: 170 bpm;
- respiratory rate: 55;
- full pulse;
- rectal temperature: 39.8 °C;
- mucous membranes: pink, CRT <1.5 seconds;
- blood pressure: 85/57 mmHg, MAP: 65 mmHg;
- dehydration: about 12%;
- pain on abdominal palpation and intestinal loop enlargement;
- hot extremities.

Chapter 3 ♦ Fluids: when and how to administer them

Laboratory tests

A blood gas analysis was performed because a disease affecting the extracellular compartment (ECF) was suspected, although it could also involve the intracellular compartment. It is important perform this test, as it guides us in the choice of fluid therapy and of a treatment for the acid-base imbalances that are most likely present.

A blood count was also performed to evaluate the hematocrit and white blood cell levels, which are useful for therapeutic and prognostic purposes.

The measurement of biochemical parameters is also useful to assess whether the organs related to the gastrointestinal system are compromised or if there is multiple organ failure. In this case, given the presence of diarrhea with blood, coagulation tests were also performed to exclude any poisoning, and a blood smear was made to evaluate platelets. A blood smear is recommended in all critically ill patients, however, since it can provide a lot of information at a very low cost (e.g., erythrocyte morphology, leukocyte count, presence of parasites). An ELISA test was also performed for the rapid diagnosis of canine parvovirus infection.

Arterial blood gas analysis

Since there was an increase in the respiratory rate and severe prostration, the effectiveness of the cardiorespiratory system in oxygenating the blood was also evaluated, for which an arterial sample from the metatarsal artery was collected. The blood gas analysis also allows oxygen parameters to be calculated and the pH, bicarbonate, carbon dioxide and electrolytes levels to be determined.

- pH: 7.38;
- $paCO_2$: 25;
- paO_2: 85;
- HCO_3^-: 15;
- BE: -9,7;
- Na^+: 134 mmol/L;
- Cl^-: 127 mmol/L;
- K^+: 3,1 mmol/L;
- lactate: 5.4 mmol/L;
- AG: 4,9;
- FiO_2: 0.21.

Clinical Case

Biochemical profile

BUN 30 mg/dL, creatinine 1.2 mg/dL, ALT 41 U/L, AST 35 U/L, total proteins 3.7 g/dL, albumin 0.9 g/dL, total bilirubin 0.5 mg/dL, GGT 14 U/L, blood glucose 78 mg/100 mL, phosphorus 5.4 mg/dL.

Complete blood count

RBC 4.9×10^{12}/L, WBC 7.3×10^{9}/L, Hct 29%, Hb 9.5 g/dL, PLT 104×10^{9}/L, neutrophils 12×10^{3}/µL, normal platelet count.

Coagulation test

In this case the PT test was performed: 8.5 seconds; the aPTT was about 27 seconds and the fibrinogen was approximately 180 mg/dL.

Interpretation of laboratory tests

The blood gas analysis showed an almost normal pH but an altered $paCO_2$, which suggested the presence of respiratory alkalosis, while bicarbonate levels indicated the presence of metabolic acidosis. Therefore, according to the traditional approach, this was a case of mixed acid-base imbalance. It was therefore necessary to decide which acid-base imbalance should be treated first so it could be done as quickly as possible. In general, the imbalance that compromises more vital functions must be treated first. Many times, treating the main problem also treats mixed acid-base imbalances. In this case, by treating circulatory failure (i.e., hypotension and peripheral vasodilation), vomiting and diarrhea, the main problems are treated.

Hypoxia was also present due to the decreased paO_2. The paO_2/FiO_2 ratio was about 405, which was indicative of an effective although suboptimal oxygenation. However, oxygen therapy was recommended given the dog's critical condition.

According to the nontraditional approach, the pH revealed mild acidemia, while severe SID acidemia (94 nmol/L) was present. At the same time there was a very high concentration of unmeasured cations; the A_{tot} helped to correct acidosis as they were reduced, and respiratory alkalosis contributed to raising the pH. The greatest contribution was given by the increase in SID (presence of unmeasured cations).

Chapter 3 ♦ Fluids: when and how to administer them

Biochemical tests showed a reduction in proteins and albumin probably due to protein-losing enteropathy caused by a lesion of the gastroenteric mucosa.
Multiple organ failure was not present, as the other biochemical parameters were normal. At that moment there was no leukopenia and lymphopenia but monitoring was required over the following days.
The coagulation tests ruled out anticoagulant rodenticide poisoning since the PT was normal while the aPTT was prolonged.
The osmolarity is calculated as follows:

$$Osm = 2 \times [Na+] + glucose\ (mg/dL)\ /18 + BUN\ (mg/dL)/2.8$$

$$Osm = (2 \times 134) + (78/18) + (30/2.8)$$

$$Osm = 283\ mOsm/L$$

Osmolarity was slightly reduced compared to normal values as a result of reduced natremia. In this case, the administration of an isotonic saline solution containing large amounts of sodium (e.g., Ringer's acetate or Normosol-R with sodium gluconate) can be useful to correct the problem.

Diagnostic tests

An X-ray (shown below) of the abdomen was taken and did not reveal the presence of foreign bodies, but intestinal loop enlargement was present.
Other lesions of the gastrointestinal tract cannot be detected with this diagnostic test. As the dog was a puppy, it was chosen to use this imaging technique to assess the presence of foreign bodies (e.g., stones, bones or fragments of wood), which is frequent in young dogs.

Daily fluid therapy

As the patient was hypotensive, with perfusion parameters that suggested a circulatory deficit, it was decided to administer a fluid bolus of Plasma-Lyte with sodium gluconate. A dose of 240 mL was delivered over 20 minutes, but this did not improve the hemodynamic condition. A second bolus was therefore administered, which was able to normalize the patient's perfusion parameters. At this point it was decided to switch to daily maintenance fluid therapy plus fluids to treat dehydration.

If the patient had not responded to fluid resuscitation, the administration of vasoactive drugs (e.g., CRI of norepinephrine) should have been considered. In this case the risk of requiring vasoactive support was high, as the hot extremities could lead to the suspicion of the presence of peripheral vasodilation and sepsis.

The recommended fluid therapy was a maintenance fluid therapy with a high SID, to attempt to correct the metabolic acidosis. In this case, daily fluid therapy consisted in the administration of Plasma-Lyte with sodium gluconate. The volume of fluids lost (12% dehydration) must also be added to the maintenance fluids.

Maintenance fluids: 2 mL/kg/hour IV, which corresponds to 24 mL/hour IV.

Dehydration: 12% of 12 kg corresponds to 1440 mL/ day, which once divided by 24 hours corresponds to 60 mL/ hour IV.

Due to the severely decreased serum albumin concentration, it was decided to simultaneously administer 5% human albumin at a dose of 20 mL/kg/day and at a rate of 2 mL/kg/hour IV. Albumin was administered for 3 consecutive days, because the serum albumin concentration remained low.

Additional therapy

The patient, in addition to 5% human albumin, was given broad-spectrum antibiotics: amoxicillin and clavulanic acid 20 mg/kg every 12 hours IV, and metronidazole 20 mg/kg every 12 hours IV. For emesis, metoclopramide was administered as a CRI at a dose of 0.02 mg/kg/hour IV; 1 gram of diosmectite every 8 hours was also administered. A nasal cannula was placed on the patient to bring the FiO_2 to 0.40. The patient was discharged on the fifth day, when he resumed eating and drinking spontaneously.

Electrolyte Disorders

Fabio Viganò, Corinna Uboldi

CHAPTER 4

Introduction

Body fluids consist of water, the solvent, and the particles dissolved in it, the solutes.

Water is the major component of body fluids and in dogs and cats it accounts for about 60% of the total body weight. It is distributed in distinct compartments, namely the intracellular compartment (intracellular fluid, ICF), which contains most of the body fluids (about 2/3) and the extracellular compartment (extracellular fluid, ECF), which contains a much smaller amount (about 1/3) (see Chapter 1). In addition to water, body fluids contain various solutes distributed differently in the two compartments (Figure 4.1). Solutes are molecules that can be dissociated into electrically charged atoms, called ions. Ions can have a positive charge (cations) or a negative charge (anions). Because of this they can conduct electrochemical energy and are called electrolytes.

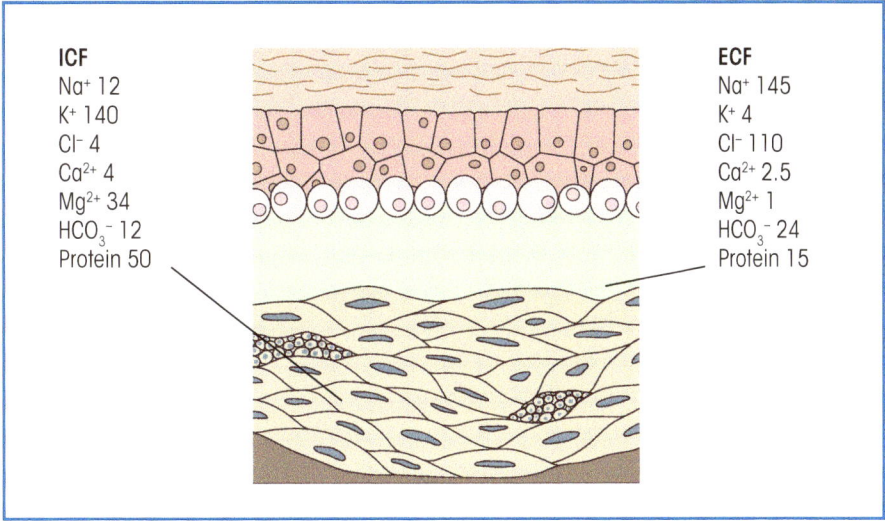

ICF
Na^+ 12
K^+ 140
Cl^- 4
Ca^{2+} 4
Mg^{2+} 34
HCO_3^- 12
Protein 50

ECF
Na^+ 145
K^+ 4
Cl^- 110
Ca^{2+} 2.5
Mg^{2+} 1
HCO_3^- 24
Protein 15

Figure 4.1 Concentration of electrolytes in the extra- and intracellular compartments. ICF, intracellular compartment; ECF, extracellular compartment.

Chapter 4 ◆ Electrolyte Disorders

Each electrolyte is characterized by a valence, which is the ability to create chemical bonds based on the magnitude of its charges. For example, sodium has one positive charge and is thus defined as monovalent, i.e., it can bind to an atom with a monovalent negative charge, such as chloride; calcium, on the other hand, has a double positive charge, can bind to two chloride atoms and for this reason it is defined as bivalent.

Electrolytes are therefore particles that dissociate into ions with a negative or positive charge as they dissolve in water. This phenomenon is called ionization. A typical example of this reaction is the dissociation of hydrochloric acid: $HCl + H_2O \leftrightarrows H3O^+ + Cl^-$.

The aqueous solution containing the electrolytes thus dissociated is able to conduct the electric current. If dissociation is complete (called quantitative) or almost complete (equilibrium to the right), the electrolytes that are free are defined as strong. If dissociation is partial, i.e., the electrolytes only have a slight tendency to dissociate and a part or most of them remain linked to the molecule from which they originated, they are defined as weak and remain largely in solution in a non-dissociated form. An example of complete dissociation of an acid, which is therefore defined as strong, is that of hydrochloric acid (HCl); an example of a strong base is sodium hydroxide (NaOH), while the chemical species that partially dissociate and are thus considered weak are carbonic acid (H_2CO_3) and ammonia (NH_3).

Electrolytes, in clinical practice, are measured in equivalents (Eq). One Eq is defined as a mole of any anion that combines with hydrogen, or a mole of any monovalent cation that can replace hydrogen in the following chemical reaction: 1 mole of H^+ + 1 mole of Cl^- = 1 mole of HCl (monovalent cation); or 1 mole of Ca^{2+} + 2 moles of Cl^- = 1 mole of $CaCl_2$ (bivalent cation).

In biological fluids, electrolyte concentrations are very diluted and for this reason milliequivalents (mEq) are generally used as a unit of measurement.

Osmosis

The different concentration of solutes between the intracellular compartment (ICF) and the extracellular compartment (ECF) is regulated by the presence of semipermeable membranes, which allow the passage of water and some solutes. The movement of water through semipermeable membranes (e.g., the cell wall membrane) creates a pressure gradient that is called osmosis. Water moves from the less concentrated to the more concentrated compartment.

If a solute is in higher concentration in a compartment, it generates a movement of water to that compartment. The measurement of the volume of displaced water is called the osmotic pressure of the solute. According to the Gibbs–Donnan effect,

Chapter 4 ◆ Electrolyte Disorders

large molecules (e.g., proteins) with a negative charge attract positive charges to their compartment and drive negatively charged molecules away. These phenomena occur with no expenditure of energy and only by osmotic gradient.

The solutes that freely cross the semipermeable membranes reach balanced concentrations on both sides of the membrane without resulting in solvent movement.

Osmotic pressure is defined as the hydrostatic pressure necessary to prevent the phenomenon of osmosis and is expressed in mmHg. It depends on the number of particles, so an increase in positive charges close to the negative charges of proteins will increase their osmotic effect. This osmotic effect of a nondiffusible colloid is called oncotic pressure and is the reason for the difference in osmotic pressure between the protein-rich plasma and the interstitial fluid.

Osmolarity and osmolality

Osmolarity is defined as the concentration of osmotically active particles in 1 liter of solution (Osm/L), while osmolality indicates the concentration of osmotically active particles in 1 kilogram of water (Osm/kg).

The osmotic activity of a solution is related to the number of particles present in it, regardless of their mass or charge. Molecules that do not dissociate, such as glucose and urea, will have a number of osmotically active particles (osmoles and milliosmoles) equal to the number of molecules in the solution, i.e., 1 millimole equals 1 milliosmole. Molecules that dissociate will produce more milliosmoles when the solutes are dissociated. For example, sodium chloride is dissociated into sodium ions and chloride ions, so 1 millimole of NaCl generates 2 milliosmoles. To have an osmotic effect, the solute must be on only one side of the semipermeable membrane. Small molecules, such as urea, are diffused freely through some membranes (e.g., the vascular membrane) and therefore do not generate an effective osmolality; conversely, if the solute is too large to cross the semipermeable membrane (e.g., proteins and vascular wall), the molecules will exert an osmotic effect.

Effective osmolality is called tonicity and refers to the ability of solutes to create an osmotic force by moving water between compartments separated by semipermeable membranes. Sodium, for example, cannot cross a semipermeable membrane such as that of the cell, and its movement is regulated by the sodium–potassium pump. This pump requires energy (ATP, adenosine triphosphate), which is obtained through oxidative phosphorylation in the mitochondria and thus requires oxygen. Because it remains outside the cell wall, sodium exerts an osmotic effect that attracts water to this compartment. Conversely, although it represents part of the dissolved solutes, urea is freely diffusible and does not produce the movement of solvent. Sodium is responsible for the tonicity of extracellular fluids, while potassium maintains the tonicity of intracellular fluids.

Chapter 4 ◆ Electrolyte Disorders

Isotonic solutions are defined as those that have the same tonicity as the body's fluids (very close to 300 mOsm), such as 0.9% NaCl. Hypotonic solutions have a lower osmolality than biological fluids, while hypertonic solutions have a higher tonicity. Sometimes the hypertonicity of a solution is incompatible with its administration through the peripheral veins, and solutions with an osmolality >600 mOsm should be administered in the central vessels (e.g., jugular vein).

The osmolality of blood can be calculated using the following formula:

$$Osm = (2 \times Na) + (BUN/2) + (glucose/18) \qquad (Equation\ 1)$$

With this formula, the osmotic pressure is calculated based mainly on the blood sodium concentration; it is not measured (see Chapter 1). In the presence of osmotically active molecules, as in hyperlipemia, the osmotic pressure calculated using the formula above may not correspond to the patient's actual osmotic pressure. However, it can detect alterations in osmotic pressure caused by hyperglycemia or azotemia, which are common in critically ill patients.

Sodium

Seventy percent of the body's sodium is found in the extracellular and intracellular fluids; it can be exchanged between these different compartments. Of this share, about 81% is found in the interstitial and transcellular fluids, 16% in plasma and 3% in the intracellular compartment. The remaining sodium is contained in the bones and is therefore difficult to use.

The need for water is detected through changes in blood tonicity, which depends on natremia. Central osmoreceptors are located in the lamina terminalis of the hypothalamus, adjacent to the third ventricular wall. Sensory cells are activated by changes in plasma osmolarity that promote water movement between the ICF and the ECF. They are also activated when an expansion in blood volume is required and during hypotension.

Osmoreceptors can activate the thirst center and the neurons of the supraoptic nucleus, which contains vasopressin that is transported to the posterior pituitary. If ECF tonicity increases, thirst and the release of ADH are stimulated; conversely, if tonicity decreases, an inhibitory effect is produced. In addition, ADH release is influenced by afferents from the brainstem, which respond to blood volume variations. The so-called "high pressure" receptors, which are located in the carotid sinus and aortic arch, are sensitive to changes in arterial blood volume, and modulate sympathetic and parasympathetic activity as well as ADH release. In the presence of hypovolemia, these receptors elicit an increase in sympathetic activity and a decrease in parasympathetic activity, which results in an increased heart rate and peripheral vasoconstriction. Increased ADH enhances vasoconstriction by acting on the smooth muscle cells and reduces diuresis, thereby promoting sodium retention. High pressure receptors are also present in the afferent arterioles of the renal glomeruli. As they detect changes in perfusion, these receptors modulate the production of renin. For example, when perfusion of the renal afferent arterioles is reduced due to hypovolemia, juxtaglomerular cells increase renin secretion. Renin converts angiotensinogen into angiotensin I, which is in turn converted into angiotensin II; subsequently, by enzymatic cascade, angiotensin III and IV are produced. Angiotensin II causes arteriolar vasoconstriction and stimulates thirst and ADH release at the central nervous system level. At the kidney level, preferential vasoconstriction of the efferent arteriole occurs, which aims to hinder the outflow of blood from the glomerulus in order to increase the pressure and maintain the filtration pressure. Finally, angiotensin II and III stimulates the secretion of aldosterone from the adrenal cortex, which promotes sodium reabsorption in the distal tubule (Figure 4.2).

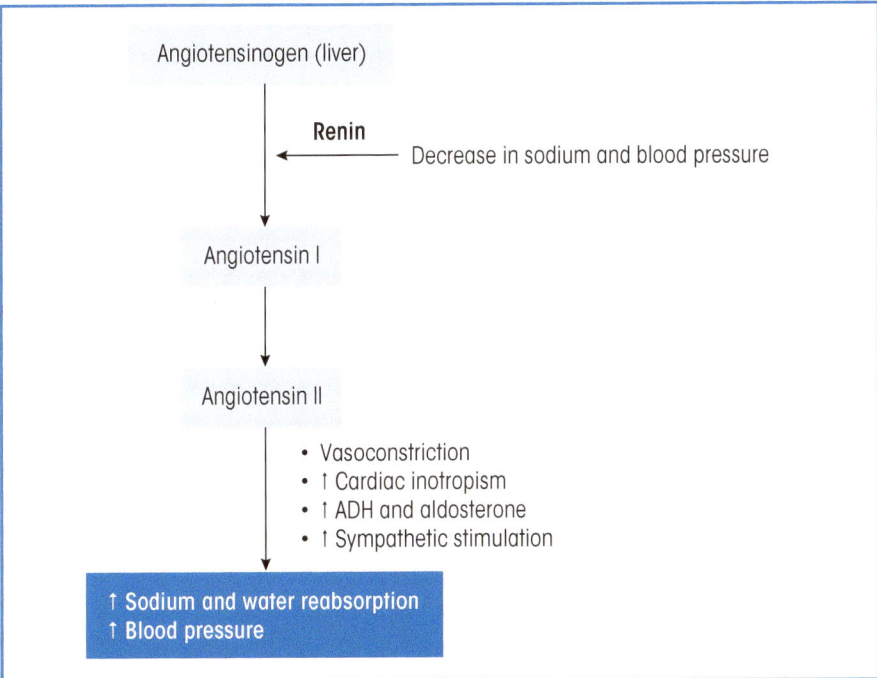

Figure 4.2 Renin–angiotensin–aldosterone system in sodium and water reabsorption.

Chapter 4 ◆ Electrolyte Disorders

The ADH released enters the circulation and reaches the renal peritubular capillaries, where it diffuses towards the tubules and acts by binding to the V2 receptors of the collecting tubule cells, which are found at their basal surface, facing the interstitium. This binding induces important cellular events, including the synthesis and expression of new channels for water reabsorption (aquaporins) on the cell surface facing the tubular lumen. This results in water retention and a decrease in ECF tonicity.

The amount of sodium excreted in urine depends on glomerular filtration (amount of filtered sodium that reaches the kidney) and its tubular reabsorption (sodium saved). Glomerular filtration depends on hydrostatic pressure (difference between blood pressure and Bowman's capsule), which induces filtration, and the oncotic pressure of albumin, which hinders it. Fifty percent of the tubular reabsorption of sodium occurs at the proximal tubule, where there are Na–H exchangers between the cells and tubule. Protons are eliminated in exchange for sodium, which passes from the lumen into the tubular cell. This exchange is favored, indirectly, by the sodium–potassium pump, which is found on the basolateral side of the cell and pumps $3Na^+$ into the interstitium and only $2K^+$ into the cell. Due to the net loss of positive charges, the intracellular potential is more negative than the tubular fluid and favors the entry of sodium.

During hypovolemia, a reduction in glomerular perfusion and in pressure in the capillaries of the afferent arteriole surrounding the proximal tubule favors oncotic reabsorption and hydrostatic absorption. The opposite effect occurs in case of hypervolemia.

The loop of Henle reabsorbs about 45% of the filtered sodium. At the level of its ascending branch, the tubular wall becomes impermeable to water but maintains its permeability to solutes. A Na–K–2Cl cotransporter acts at this level to transport chloride inside the cell together with sodium. Sodium is also passively reabsorbed by the thin ascending branch of the loop. Reabsorption by the loop of Henle is stimulated by sympathetic activity, ADH release, and reduced blood flow in the medullary capillaries.

The distal tubule, on the other hand, reabsorbs 3% of the filtered sodium. Sodium enters together with chloride from the luminal side and is actively transferred into the interstitium by the Na–K pump located on the basal side.

About 2% of sodium is reabsorbed in the collecting tubule. The main cells absorb sodium from the tubular lumen and release it into the interstitium at their basal side, where it is exchanged for potassium thanks to an ionic pump that is activated by aldosterone and keeps the intracellular concentration of sodium low.

Sodium is then eliminated mainly by the kidney, which regulates its excretion according to the needs of the body and thus controls the amount of sodium in the extracellular fluid and, consequently, the blood volume. Another route of excretion, but of lesser magnitude, is elimination through feces.

Chapter 4 ◆ Electrolyte Disorders

Hyponatremia

Hyponatrema is a condition characterized by a low sodium concentration (dog <145 mEq/L, cat <150 mEq/L) that frequently, but not always, causes hyposmolality. In hyponatremic patients it is necessary to first determine the osmolality of the ECF by calculating, or rather measuring, the osmolality of plasma. The following three conditions can be associated with hyponatremia:

- *Hyponatremia with normal osmolality* (290–310 mOsm/kg): it is also called pseudohyponatremia, as the presence of a high amount of lipids and proteins artificially alters tonicity. In these patients, it is not necessary to correct hyponatremia but the pathological process that causes hyperproteinemia and hyperlipidemia.
- *Hyponatremia with increased plasma osmolality* (>310 mOsm/kg): this situation occurs, for example, when there are other molecules in addition to sodium capable of increasing blood tonicity, as in hyperosmolar syndromes (e.g., uncontrolled diabetes mellitus, administration of mannitol). Because glucose is an effective osmole, i.e., it can draw water from the intracellular into the extracellular compartment, it causes a reduction in sodium concentration due to dilution. It is therefore not a true hyponatremia, but the consequence of sodium dilution. As in the previous case, it is not necessary to correct hyponatremia but the pathological process that causes it (e.g., treatment of diabetes).
- *Hyponatremia with reduced plasma osmolality* (<290 mOsm/kg): it requires determination of whether the patient is normovolemic, hypovolemic, or hypervolemic. In order to identify which condition is associated with hyponatremia, the clinical history should be taken (presence of vomiting, diarrhea, tachypnea, administration of diuretics, or drugs that promote diuresis), the clinical parameters used to assess the hydration status should be evaluated (skin turgor through the skin fold test, skin edema, presence of skin fovea, dryness of the mucous membranes—especially the oral mucous membranes—, CRT, pulse, ectasia of the jugular vein, presence of a jugular pulse, ascites, blood pressure, disappeared heart sounds, and dulling of breathing sounds), and the hematocrit and total plasma proteins should be measured (Figure 4.3);
  - Hyponatremia with normovolemia: it is caused by inappropriate ADH secretion due to abnormal vasopressin production. The causes can be:
    - Psychogenic polydipsia, a condition seen especially in large dogs after a stressful event, or in hyperactive dogs kept in a very small place. It has not been demonstrated in cats [1].
    - Syndrome of inappropriate antidiuretic hormone secretion (SIADH): it is rare in dogs and is reported in association with heartworm disease, carcinoma, neoplasms of the hypothalamus, granulomatous meningoencephalitis, hydrocephalus, and idiopathic causes [2].

Chapter 4 ◆ Electrolyte Disorders

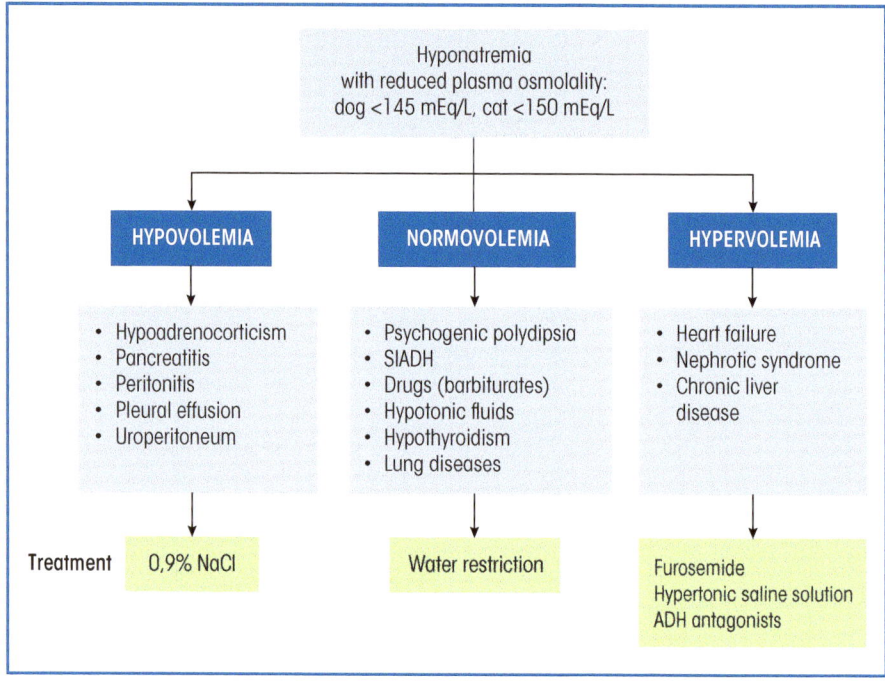

Figure 4.3 Causes and therapy of hyponatremia with reduced blood osmolality.

- Administration of barbiturates, nitrous oxide, narcotics, isoproterenol.
- Use of hypotonic fluids [3].
- Lung diseases (ARDS, bacterial pneumonia).
- Hypothyroidism.
- Hyponatremia with hypovolemia: a typical example is hypoadrenocorticism [4], which causes a loss of NaCl in urine and a reduction in the ECF volume, which in turn stimulates vasopressin release and impairs water excretion. Other causes are the administration of diuretics and fluid losses secondary to vomiting and diarrhea. Three events leading to hyponatremia can occur:
  - Hypovolemia causes a reduction in glomerular filtration resulting in reduced water excretion.
  - Hypovolemia stimulates the release of vasopressin, which leads to an increase in its concentration in plasma and impairs water excretion.
  - There is not enough water available to meet the patient's needs. Other causes are fluid leakage during pancreatitis, peritonitis, uroperitoneum, pleural effusion.

Chapter 4 ◆ Electrolyte Disorders

– *Hyponatremia with hypervolemia*: a condition found in patients with edema or ascites resulting from heart failure, severe chronic liver disease and nephrotic syndrome. It can be due to three alterations:
  – Activation of the renin–angiotensin–aldosterone system, which leads to reduced renal perfusion and thus to increased sodium retention by the kidney and reduced water excretion.
  – Vasopressin release with reduced water excretion.
  – Activation of the kidney's intrinsic mechanism of sodium retention in nephrotic syndrome.

Clinical signs

They appear especially during acute hyponatremia. The most common are lethargy, nausea, weight gain, and vomiting. More severe signs may also occur, such as cerebral and pulmonary edema, weakness, incoordination, convulsions, stupor, and coma. Chronic hyponatremia is generally not responsible for pathognomonic signs.

Treatment

Symptomatic acute hyponatremia requires administration of 0.9% NaCl or of another solution with a high sodium concentration. The volume of solution to be administered can be calculated by measuring the patient's blood sodium concentration and subtracting it from the normal sodium concentration. The value obtained is multiplied by the body weight, as shown in the formula below (Box 4.1):

$$(140 - [Na^+]_p) \times kg \times 0.3 = Na^+ \text{ deficiency} \qquad (Equation\ 2)$$

The sodium deficiency thus obtained must be divided by the sodium concentration of the chosen solution, as shown in the following formula:

$$Na^+ \text{ deficiency}/[Na^+] \text{ of the solution} = \text{volume, in liters,}$$
$$\text{of solution to be administered}$$
$$(Equation\ 3)$$

The formula below can be used to calculate the duration of administration of the solution:

$$(140 - [Na^+]_p)/0.5 = \text{number of hours of fluid therapy} \qquad (Equation\ 4)$$

In chronic hyponatremia, to avoiding correcting the blood sodium too quickly when using solutions other than 0.9% NaCl, the sodium deficiency can be calculated as follows:

Chapter 4 ◆ Electrolyte Disorders

> **Box 4.1**   **Treatment of acute hyponatremia**
>
> **Acute hyponatremia: dog <145 mEq/L, cat <150 mEq/L**
>
> - $(140 - [Na^+]p) \times kg \times 0.3 = Na^+$ deficit
> - Na+ deficit/$[Na^+]$ of the solution = volume in liters of solution to be administered
> - $(140 - [Na^+]_p) / 0.5$ = number of hours of infusion
> - Maximum correction speed: 0.5 mEq/hour, better over 48–72 hours
> - Chronic hyponatremia: $[Na^+]_p - Na^+$ in the fluid = Na^+ to be added to 1 L of solution
> - Pure water losses: patient weight (kg) $\times 0.6 \times [([Na^+]_p / [Na^+]_n) - 1]$ = water deficit in liters
>
> $[Na^+]_p$, natremia of the patient; $[Na^+]_n$, normal natremia.

$[Na^+]_p - Na^+$ in the fluid = Na^+ to be added to 1 L of solution   *(Equation 5)*

When the patient has lost pure water, such a deficit can be calculated as follows:

Patient's weight (kg) $\times 0.6 \times [([Na^+]_p / [Na^+]_n) - 1]$ = water deficit in liters

(Equation 6)

    Correction should be progressive, as cells produce other osmotically active molecules to control the imbalance, which are slowly eliminated. This mechanism allows cells to adapt to the transport of sodium, potassium, and other solutes from inside to outside the cell. The presence of these solutes lowers intracellular osmolality and slows down the entry of water into the intracellular environment, thus reducing the extent of edema.

    The maximum rate of correction of hyponatremia should be 0.5 mEq/L/hour (10–12 mEq/L/hour) to reduce the risk of central pontine myelinolysis, an irreversible brain condition that may appear approximately 3–4 days after treatment. As an indication, 10 mEq/L should be corrected in the first 24 hours, and a maximum of 18 mEq/L in the first 48 hours. Hyponatremia should ideally be corrected over 48–72 hours.

    In overhydrated patients with cerebral edema, solutions containing large amounts of sodium can be combined with the administration of natriuretic diuretics such as

Chapter 4 ◆ Electrolyte Disorders

furosemide in order to achieve faster correction. Symptomatic chronic hyponatremia requires the same treatment.

During the correction of hyponatremia, especially if it is rapid and hyponatremia is severe, sodium and, if possible, chloride and potassium levels should be monitored every 2–4 hours until these values normalize. The patient's vital parameters and neurological status should be assessed every 8 hours, while the acid–base balance should be evaluated every 12–24 hours.

In patients with chronic and asymptomatic hyponatremia, correction should occur slowly since rapid correction is more dangerous than the disorder itself. In these cases, the administration of saline solutions that are hypernatremic relative to plasma must therefore be avoided.

Rapid correction (in 38 hours) of chronic hyponatremia, such as that caused by trichuriasis, can lead to neurological signs such as lethargy, nausea, ataxia, hypermetria, and tetraparesis [5].

Patients with chronic hyponatremia (normovolemic or hypervolemic) and with heart failure can be treated with diuretics and ACE inhibitors, which, by improving cardiac output, reducing preload and afterload, and decreasing vasopressin secretion, increase water excretion and can improve and correct hyponatremia.

Hypovolemic patients need correction with solutions containing high sodium concentrations, such as 0.9% NaCl.

Research is underway to establish the efficacy of antagonists of the arginine-vasopressin receptors (vaptans), V2 receptors (lixivaptan, tolvaptan, satavaptan) and V2 and V1 receptors (conivaptan), which increase water excretion, thereby normalizing natremia in patients with normovolemia or hypervolemia. Conivaptan is added to a 5% dextrose solution and administered intravenously as a constant rate infusion, while tolvaptan, lixivaptan and satavaptan are administered orally.

In human patients these drugs have minimal side effects (thirst and dry mouth) and minimize the risk of developing neurological symptoms in the days following the correction of hyponatremia. They correct natremia in 24 hours.

Hypernatremia

Hypernatremia is defined as a sodium concentration >160 mEq/L. Hypernatremia can be due to water deficiencies such as:
- *Central diabetes insipidus*, due to no or insufficient release of vasopressin, responsible for the formation of urine with a low specific gravity (decreased urinary concentration). The causes can be of neurological origin—such as primary pituitary neoplasia, meningioma, head trauma, pituitary surgery, and metastatic-parasitic-inflammatory lesions—or of idiopathic origin in young dogs. The clini-

cal signs are polyuria and polydipsia, with the animal constantly seeking water; weight loss; and neurological signs.
- Hypernatremia of renal origin responsible for water loss. It can be due to insensitivity of the renal tubules to vasopressin, which has been reported in Huskies in which it has a genetic origin, or result from diabetes mellitus, pyometra, hyper- or hypoadrenocorticism, hyperthyroidism in the cat, and congenital or acquired nephropathies.

The diagnosis of both forms can be achieved through urine examination, water deprivation tests, and plasma vasopressin dosage. Treatment involves the administration of vasopressin/desmopressin for the central form, and thiazide diuretics as well as a low-sodium diet for the nephrogenic form.

Other causes of hypernatremia are:
- *severely increased ambient temperature*;
- *high fever*;
- *inadequate access to water*;
- *postobstructive diuresis*;
- *excessive fluid loss due to extrarenal causes* (vomiting, diarrhea, small bowel obstruction, peritonitis, pancreatitis, and burns) and renal causes (administration of diuretics, mannitol, chronic kidney disease, acute renal failure, and diabetes mellitus);
- *primary adipsia*, congenital in the Miniature Schnauzer;
- *administration of hypertonic fluids*, e.g., sodium bicarbonate, hypertonic saline;
- *administration of drugs* that can cause diuresis such as gentamicin and amphotericin B, furosemide, corticosteroids, mannitol;
- *glycosuria*;
- *ketonuria*;
- *hyperadrenocorticism*;
- *hyperaldosteronism*.

Clinical signs

The clinical signs are numerous and not always pathognomonic: anorexia, depression, vomiting and diarrhea, muscle weakness, behavioral alterations and disorientation, pulmonary edema, tachycardia, polyuria, hyperthermia.

When the sodium concentration exceeds 170 mEq/L, neurological signs appear such as epileptic seizures, coma, stupor, and ataxia. The more severe the signs and with neurological manifestations, the more the imbalance has arisen quickly; this is due to dehydration of the brain cells, which alters their function.

Chapter 4 ◆ Electrolyte Disorders

Treatment

Acute hypernatremia should be promptly corrected with infusion of a 0.9% saline solution. In some cases, fluid resuscitation with 0.9% NaCl is necessary and involves the administration of 20 ml/kg IV over 15–20 minutes; 2–3 boluses can be repeated if necessary.

In severe forms of chronic hypernatremia, or when the duration of hypernatriemia is unknown (it must be considered chronic until proven otherwise), the correction of blood sodium should be gradual and achieved with 0,9% NaCl to avoid excessively rapid changes in blood osmolarity, as they carry a risk of neurological damage. In these cases, the following formula may be used:

$$[Na^+] \text{ of the patient} - [Na^+] \text{ of the fluid} = Na^+ \text{ to be added to 1 L of water}$$

(Equation 7)

The solution to be infused can be prepared with water for injection and hypertonic saline solution, or 5% dextrose solution and hypertonic saline solution.

In acute forms of hypernatremia, rapid correction is generally well tolerated. However, the correction rate should be less than 0.5 mEq/L/hour. Monitoring of natremia should be performed every 4–6 hours. Complete correction should be achieved in 48–72 hours. In these cases, the following formula can be used:

$$([Na^+] \text{ of the patient}/[Na^+] \text{ normal} - 1) \times (0.6 \times \text{kg patient}) =$$
$$\text{L of isotonic saline solution}$$

(Equation 8)

The maximum correction rate can be 1 mEq/L/hour if the blood sodium concentration is less than 180 mEq/L. When blood sodium is greater than 180 mEq/L, the correction rate should be 0.5 mEq/L/hour to reduce the risk of cerebral edema and neurological damage. When fluid overload occurs, furosemide may be used to reduce blood volume and natremia.

Monitoring can be performed by assessing the following parameters:
- natremia, every 4 hours in severe forms and every 6–12 hours otherwise;
- physical examination: temperature, heart and respiratory rates, pulse, color and hydration of the mucous membranes, water retention (weigh the patient twice a day), blood pressure and urine output every 8 hours;
- neurological status (Glasgow coma scale) every 8 hours;
- hydration status every 12 hours (e.g., by measuring hematocrit, total proteins and physical signs); acid–base status every 12–24 hours.

Chapter 4 ◆ Electrolyte Disorders

Potassium

Potassium is an essential element for most living organisms, and it is present in organic fluids in its ionized form (K^+) or bound to nondiffusible anions such as proteins. Muscle tissue is particularly rich in potassium (it contains about 2200 mEq). Ninety-seven percent of potassium is found in the ICF at a concentration of about 160 mEq/L, compared to 3.5–5 mEq/L in the ECF. These concentrations are maintained predominantly by the sodium–potassium (Na–K) pump, which is powered by ATP and can be found in the outer plasma membrane of the cell. The Na–K pump keeps potassium inside the cell and expels sodium. The factors that regulate potassium movements between the ECF and ICF are:

- Acid–base balance: during metabolic acidosis, excess hydrogen ions are buffered by entering the intracellular environment, which breaks electroneutrality. To restore electroneutrality, potassium is drawn into the extracellular compartment. For each 0.1 pH reduction, potassium increases by 0.7 mmol/L. The situation is slightly different in respiratory acidosis, where the increase in potassium is about 0.1 mmol/L lower for each decimal reduction in pH. During metabolic or respiratory alkalosis, on the other hand, there is a reduction in hydrogen ions in the intracellular environment, so potassium enters the cell to compensate for the loss of positive charges. For each decimal increase in pH there is a reduction in potassium of 0.3 mmol/L.
- Pancreatic hormones: insulin activates the Na–K pump and causes cellular uptake of potassium in exchange for sodium, which exits the cell; this therefore decreases the blood potassium concentration. Glucagon, by opposite mechanisms, increases the blood potassium concentration.
- Catecholamines: they act by stimulating ß receptors which, like insulin, activate the Na–K pump by promoting the entry of K^+ into the cell. Thanks to this mechanism, ß-agonists, such as salbutamol, can be useful in the treatment of hyperkalemia.
- Aldosterone: it acts by directly activating the Na–K pump or by promoting the entry of sodium into the cell.
- Osmolality: hyperosmolality causes an extracellular flow of water, which carries with it potassium in the amount of 0.6 mmol/L for each increase of 10 mOsm/kg.
- Cellular necrosis: it may be produced by many causes (e.g., rhabdomyolysis, hemolysis, burns and tumor lysis) and induces potassium leakage.
- Exercise: physical effort promotes the release of potassium, but progressive training enhances the activity of the Na–K pump by increasing the ability of the myocytes to retain the cation.

Chapter 4 ◆ Electrolyte Disorders

The potassium contained in the ICF is essential for maintaining the osmotic balance and electric potential of the cell membrane. In addition, it is essential for protein synthesis and cell growth.

Ninety percent of potassium is excreted by the kidneys. It is freely filtered by the glomerulus and reabsorbed in the ascending loop of the proximal tubule. Only 25% of the filtered potassium reaches the distal tubule, where it is excreted or reabsorbed. The main regulators of renal excretion of potassium are aldosterone, vasopressin, hyperkalemia, increased anions in the tubular fluid, metabolic alkalosis, and increased tubular flow. Conversely, factors that inhibit renal excretion of potassium are hypokalemia, metabolic acidosis, and reduced tubular flow. The remaining 10% of potassium is excreted in the proximal and distal colon, where, under hormonal influence, sodium reabsorption and potassium excretion take place. The intestinal loss of potassium is limited under normal conditions, but it becomes constant during diarrhea and is an important route of excretion in case of chronic kidney disease.

Hypokalemia

When hypokalemia is diagnosed (dog <3.4 mEq/L, cat <2.9 mEq/L), it is important to establish whether it is due to pseudohypokalemia, hypokalemia from redistribution, extrarenal potassium losses or renal potassium losses:
- *Pseudohypokalemia*: blood samples with marked leukocytosis stored for hours at room temperature can produce a false hypokalemia, because leukocytes incorporate plasma potassium. The administration of insulin, hypokalemic fluids or albuterol, which induce an increase in the entry of potassium into the cell, may also be responsible for false hypokalemia.
- *Redistributive hypokalemia*: it can be due to the movement of potassium into the cells during metabolic alkalosis; to increased ß$_2$-adrenergic activity in head trauma; or to intoxication by barium, which blocks potassium channels and thus inhibits the exit of potassium from the cell.
- *Extrarenal losses*: severe diarrhea, protobstructive diuresis, polyuria with polydipsia, refeeding syndrome (caused by increased insulin secretion).
- *Renal losses*: associated with states of acidosis (e.g, during diabetic ketoacidosis), states of alkalosis (e.g., hyperaldosteronism), administration of loop diuretics (furosemide and thiazide diuretics), and severe emesis with chloride depletion.

Clinical signs
The appearance of clinical signs depends on the concentration of potassium:
- If K <3 mmol/L, the clinical signs will be muscle weakness, lethargy, atony, ileum, urinary retention, inability to concentrate urine, myocardial depression, polyuria and polydipsia, and muscle cramps.

Chapter 4 ◆ Electrolyte Disorders

- If K <1.5 mmol/L, very severe signs will develop such as cardiac and respiratory arrest; in the cat, ventroflexion of the head is frequently seen.

Hypokalemia, regardless of its severity, may be responsible for supraventricular and ventricular arrhythmias.

Treatment

Patients in a state of hypovolemic shock require fluid resuscitation with balanced crystalloids (e.g., Ringer's lactate or Plasma-Lyte with sodium gluconate).

Potassium replacement therapy can be provided following the indications obtained empirically (Table 4.1). In humans, supplementation may not take into account the concentration of potassium in the balanced crystalloid used.

The maximum rate of infusion of KCl is 0.5 mEq/kg/hour when administered intravenously; the oral dose may be doubled.

In these patients, monitoring is very important and involves the determination of potassium every 12–24 hours. During the correction of severe hypokalemia, it is advisable to perform continuous electrocardiographic monitoring. The patient's vital signs (at least the heart rate, pulse, CRT, mucous membrane color and respiratory rate) should be assessed every 8–12 hours (values must be written down) and a blood gas analysis should be performed every 12–24 hours (Box 4.2).

Hyperkalemia

Hyperkalemia (>5 mEq/L) may be caused by potassium redistribution or it may be secondary to impaired potassium excretion.

In the first case, it may result from metabolic acidosis, respiratory acidosis, treatment with betablockers or aldosterone inhibitor drugs (e.g., ACE inhibitors), KCl administration, parenteral nutrition, snakebite poisoning, hypertonic states, and malignant hyperthermia. Reduced potassium excretion may be due to urethral obstruction, severe tissue trauma, bladder rupture, thoracoabdominal effusions, reperfusion injury, infections, decreased aldosterone levels or lack of tubular response to aldosterone in adrenocortical insufficiency, hypoinsulinemia (metabolic ketoacidosis), tumor lysis, heat stroke, drugs (e.g., spironolactone, trimethoprim, heparin, triamterene, NSAIDs, cyclosporine, tacrolimus, amiloride, ACE inhibitors), or primary and secondary kidney disease with CKD. Trichuriasis, duodenal perforations and salmonellosis can also cause hyperkalemia.

False hyperkalemia, called pseudohyperkalemia, may also be seen, and can be caused by the use of hemolytic samples, marked thrombocytosis, and severe leukocytosis.

Chapter 4 ◆ Electrolyte Disorders

Table 4.1 Potassium supplementation per liter of solution

[K⁺] mEq/L	KCl per liter of solution	Maximum infusion rate (mL/kg/hour)
3.6–5.0	20	24
3.1–3.5	30	16
2.6–3.0	40	11
2.1–2.5	60	8
<2.0	80	6

Box 4.2 — Treatment of potassium imbalances

Hypokalemia correction: dog <3.4 mEq/L, cat <2.9 mEq/L

[K⁺] mEq/L	KCl per liter of solution	Maximum speed infusion (mL/kg/hour)
3.6–5.0	20	24
3.1–3.5	30	16
2.6–3.0	40	11
2.1–2.5	60	8
<2.0	80	6

Maximum correction rate: 0.5 mL/kg/hour

Correction of hyperkalemia: >7.5 mEq/L

Onset of effect

1) 10% calcium gluconate: 50–100 mg/kg IV over 10 minutes — Onset 2–5 min / Offset 20–30 min
2) Regular insulin, 0.55–1.1 IU/kg IV, followed by 1–2 g of 25% glucose for each IU of insulin; then administer 5% glucose solution — Onset <30 min
3) 25% glucose, 0.7–1 g/kg IV over 3–5 min — Onset <1 hour
4) NaHCO₃ 1–2 mEq/kg IV in slow infusion — Onset 30 min
5) Terbutaline 0.01 mg/kg IV in slow infusion — Onset 20–40 min

Monitor potassium every 8 hours. If treatments are ineffective: hemodialysis

Chapter 4 ◆ Electrolyte Disorders

In the presence of hyperkalemia, other emergency diagnostic investigations should be performed, such as measurement of the hematocrit, total proteins, blood sugar, azotemia, and serum creatinine concentration; assessment of the acid–base status; and continuous electrocardiographic monitoring.

Clinical signs

When hyperkalemia is >7.5 mEq/L, very severe clinical signs may appear, such as abnormal mentation (depressed), muscle weakness, loss of appetite, bradycardia, and possible cardiac arrest. Continuous electrocardiographic monitoring should be performed in patients diagnosed with hyperkalemia, because potassium values between 5.5 and 7.5 mEq/L cause the appearance of narrow and peaked T waves, prolonged QRS complexes, reduced R waves, and ST depression. The severity of electrocardiographic alterations is subjective, and these alterations may appear even with modest variations in potassium. When potassium is >7.5 mEq/L, it is possible to see the disappearance of P waves, atrial standstill, sine-wave rhythm, biphasic QRS complexes, ventricular flutter, ventricular fibrillation, and ventricular asystole (Figure 4.4).

Treatment

Patients in a state of shock are given fluid resuscitation with 0.9% NaCl. Hyperkalemia can be treated with the administration of 10% calcium gluconate at a dose of

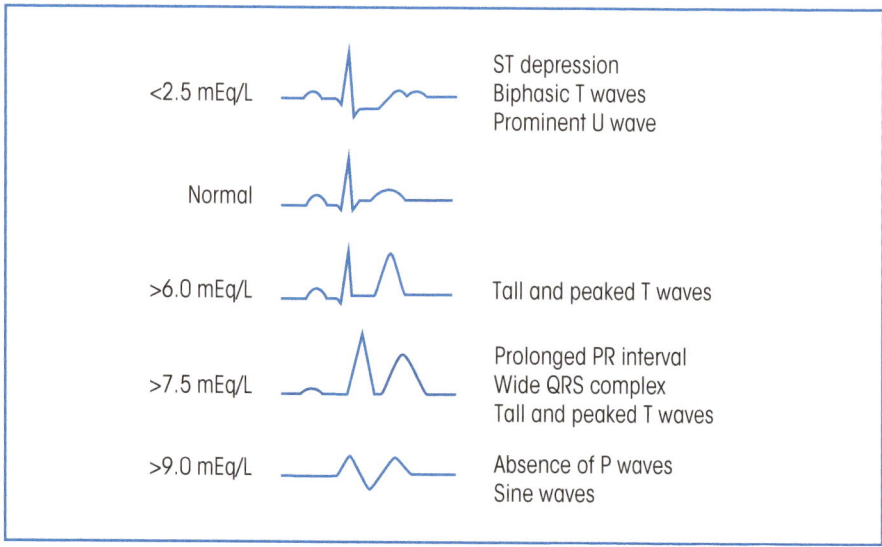

Figure 4.4 Alterations in potassium and electrocardiographic tracing

Chapter 4 ◆ Electrolyte Disorders

50–100 mg/kg IV over 10 minutes (onset 2–5 min, offset 20–30 min). This should be done under close continuous electrocardiographic monitoring because calcium gluconate can cause severe bradycardia and, if administered too quickly, cardiac arrest. Hyperkalemia can also be treated with regular insulin administration at a dose of 0.55–1.1 IU/kg IV, followed by 1–2 g of 25% dextrose for each IU of insulin; a 5% dextrose solution is therefore administered and blood sugar monitored (every 2–4 hours). Onset is less than 30 minutes. If hyperkalemia is associated with metabolic acidosis and renal failure, sodium bicarbonate at a dose of 1–2 mEq/kg IV may be administered as a slow infusion over approximately 15 minutes. This last procedure is to be avoided in hypocalcemic patients. Other treatments involve the use of 25% dextrose at a dose of 0.7–1 g/kg IV over 3–5 min (onset <1 hour), or terbutaline at a dose of 0.01 mg/kg IV as a slow infusion (onset 20–40 min).

After correcting hyperkalemia, it is necessary to treat the cause, and then to control metabolic acidosis and promote diuresis. If the above treatments are not effective, it will be necessary to resort to hemodialysis. Patients should be monitored as follows: measurement of potassium after 30 minutes from the end of the chosen protocol, to allow it to be redistributed, and then every 8–24 hours, and a blood gas analysis every 12–24 hours (see Box 4.2).

Calcium

Ninety-eight percent of body calcium is found in the bones in form of hydroxyapatite; 1% is found in plasma and the remaining 1% in the extracellular and intracellular fluids. In the extracellular fluid, calcium plays a crucial role in neuromuscular excitation processes, while in the intracellular fluid it is essential in some enzymatic reactions and during cell division. It also conditions the activity of certain hormones (e.g., calcitonin and parathyroid hormone).

Plasma calcium can be found in free (ionized) form, bound to albumin (about 40%) or bound to anions (in a small percentage, 5–10%) such as citrate, phosphate, and bicarbonate (Figure 4.5). The binding with albumin is pH-dependent: during metabolic alkalosis, proteins release hydrogen ions to compensate for metabolic alkalosis and instead fix calcium, thereby reducing its presence in ionized form. The opposite phenomenon occurs during metabolic acidosis.

The absorption of calcium takes place partly in the small intestine, with active transport thanks to the stimulation induced by vitamin D, and partly at the renal level, thanks to the activity of the parathyroid hormone (PTH). At the renal level, 50–60% of calcium is reabsorbed by the proximal tubular cells, down the electrochemical gradient, while the remaining 40% is reabsorbed in the distal tubule and

Chapter 4 ◆ Electrolyte Disorders

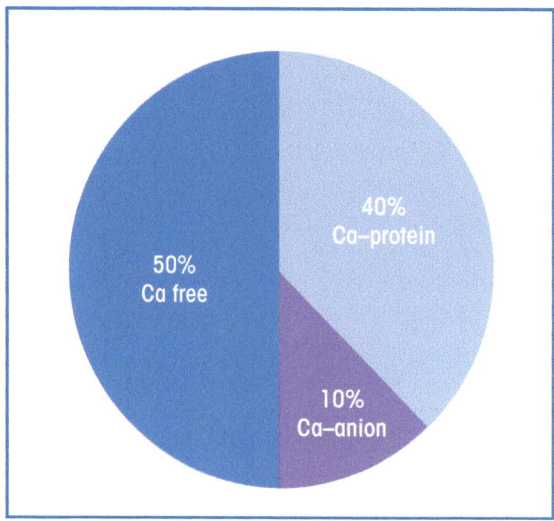

Figure 4.5 Distribution of calcium in plasma.

collecting ducts through active sodium-dependent reabsorption. This mechanism of calcium reabsorption plays a crucial role in states of hypercalcemia induced by severe dehydration. Indeed, severe dehydration stimulates the tubular reabsorption of calcium together with sodium, leading to a state of hypercalcemia. This is why appropriate fluid therapy is essential in states of hypercalcemia. Calcium from the diet is absorbed by the intestine and transported by blood to all the tissues, but more especially the bones, where the amount absorbed must be comparable to the amount released by the bones in the blood, so as to keep the circulating pool of calcium stable. This mechanism and renal tubular reabsorption constitute the actual homeostatic regulation systems of serum calcium concentration, the proper functioning of which depends on PTH, vitamin D and calcitonin.

The most powerful stimulus of PTH secretion is the reduction of ionized calcium, detected by specific membrane receptors on parathyroid cells. PTH counteracts hypocalcemia by stimulating bone resorption through osteoclast activation, tubular calcium reabsorption, and the production of renal 1-α hydroxylase, which activates vitamin D.

Calcitonin is produced by the thyroid, thymus, adrenal glands and pituitary gland. Its synthesis is stimulated by hypercalcemia, and its main function is to inhibit bone resorption. Vitamin D is formed by the action of UV sunlight and must undergo two hydroxylations to be activated, one in the liver and the other in the kidney. Its production is increased in the presence of calcium, phosphorus or vitamin D deficiency. Its main function is to increase the intestinal absorption of calcium and stimulate the

Chapter 4 ◆ Electrolyte Disorders

reabsorption of phosphorus. In the bone, vitamin D promotes the mineralization of the organic matrix and stimulates the differentiation of monocytes into osteoclasts, thus favoring the mobilization of calcium and phosphorus from the bone.

Hypocalcemia

Hypocalcemia (dog <5.0 mg/dL, cat <4.5 mg/dL) is defined as a reduction in the blood calcium level in the presence of a normal concentration of serum albumin.

The main causes of hypocalcemia are:
- *Renal failure* with impaired activation of vitamin D and a consequent reduction in the intestinal absorption of calcium. Chronic kidney disease also causes a state of hyperphosphatemia due to reduced glomerular filtration. Excess phosphorus binds to calcium and forms complexes that are subsequently removed from the cells of the reticuloendothelial system, causing hypocalcemia.
- *Insufficient PTH production* due to hypoparathyroidism (insufficient production by the parathyroid glands), caused by neoplasms, inflammation, or amyloid infiltration.
- *Acute pancreatitis*: calcium is sequestered in the necrotic tissue.
- *Paraneoplastic hypocalcemia* from osteoblastic metastases of some carcinomas (e.g., prostate and mammary carcinomas), due to the chelation of calcium by phosphates and lactates released in tissue necrosis.
- *Anticonvulsant drugs*.
- *Intoxication by ethylene glycol*, the metabolites of which chelate calcium.
- *Sepsis and ARDS*: the combination of a high concentration of proinflammatory cytokines and a high amount of lactate may cause hypocalcemia [6].
- *Puerperal eclampsia*, which occurs in the *postpartum* period (1–4 days postpartum) and during lactation.

Clinical signs

The most common signs of hypocalcemia are fasciculations, muscle tremors, facial rubbing, muscle cramping, stiff gait, and behavioral changes such as disorientation, hypersensitivity to stimuli, aggression, excitability, or restlessness. Lethargy, anorexia, pyrexia, and prolapse of the third eyelid may occasionally appear in cats, as well as, in dogs and cats, posterior and anterior cataracts, tachycardia and electrocardiographic alterations (prolongated QT interval), polyuria and polydipsia, and, in severe forms, even cardiorespiratory arrest.

Canine eclampsia manifests with neurological signs such as ataxia, tremors, myoclonus, tachypnea and tachycardia, breathlessness, pyrexia, and seizures without loss of consciousness. In severe forms, death from cerebral edema and respiratory depression may occur.

Chapter 4 ◆ Electrolyte Disorders

Treatment

Once hypocalcemia has been diagnosed, it is important to determine if it is associated with hypoalbuminemia or hypoproteinemia, as in these cases calcium should not be administered but hypoalbuminemia corrected. The concentration of PTH should then be measured to determine if the imbalance is PTH-dependent (if PTH is present in a normal concentration, hypocalcemia does not have a hormonal origin; see above).

Once the cause of hypocalcemia has been identified, it should be treated as early as possible. Blood calcium levels are corrected by administering 10% calcium gluconate as a slow infusion (over 15–20 minutes) at a dose of 0.5–1.5 mL/kg IV, or as a continuous infusion at a dose of 5–15 mg/kg/hour (Box 4.3). Another therapeutic option is the administration a continuous infusion of 10% calcium hydrochloride at a dose of 5–15 mg/kg/hour. This salt should only be administered intravenously because it is irritant and its extravasation causes perivasculitis.

Administration should be discontinued if bradycardia, QT-interval shortening, skin necrosis, or mineralization appears. To avoid the side effects of therapy, it is necessary to perform continuous electrocardiographic monitoring throughout the treatment and assess the acid–base and electrolyte balance every 12–24 hours, as well as vital signs every 8–12 hours.

Oral therapy is preferred in chronic hypocalcemia and consists in the administration of:
- calcium bicarbonate, 25–50 mg/kg/day;
- calcium lactate, 25–50 mg/kg/day;
- calcium chloride 27.2%, 25–50 mg/kg/day (may cause gastritis);
- 10% calcium gluconate, 25–50 mg/kg/day (may cause gastritis).

Box 4.3 — **Treatment of calcium imbalances**

Acute hypocalcemia: dog <5.0 mg/dL, cat <4.5 mg/dL
1) Calcium gluconate 10%: 0.5–1.5 mL/kg IV in slow infusion (over 15–20 min)
2) CRI: calcium gluconate 5–15 mg/kg/hour IV
3) CRI: calcium hydrochloride 10%: 5–15 mg/kg/hour IV
During administration, monitor with ECG.

Acute hypercalcemia: dog ≥6.0 mg/dL, cat ≥5.5 mg/dL
1) Fluid therapy with 0.9% NaCl or Plasma-Lyte with sodium gluconate
2) Furosemide 2 mg/kg IV, SC, orally, every 8–12 hours
3) Dexamethasone 0.1–0.22 mg/kg/12 hours IV, SC
4) Prednisone 1–2.2 mg/kg/12 hours IV, SC, orally
5) Calcitonin 4–6 IU/kg/8–12 hours SC for 24–48 hours
6) Biphosphonate 15 mg/kg/12–24 hours IV, orally

Chapter 4 ◆ Electrolyte Disorders

Treatment involves the simultaneous administration of vitamin D in the form of ergocalciferol (vitamin D2), initially at a dose of 4000–6000 IU/ kg/day for 5–21 days depending on the severity. In the maintenance phase, 1000–2000 IU/kg are administered once a day once a week for 1–18 weeks. Another option is the administration of calcitriol, initially at a dose of 0.2–0.3 µg/kg/day for 3–4 days, and then at 0.005–0.015 µg/kg/day for 2–14 days.

The correction is aimed at resolving the clinical signs, without necessarily achieving a normal calcium concentration so as to avoid a state of hypercalcemia and hypercalciuria, especially in patients with hypoparathyroidism.

Hypercalcemia

Hypercalcemia (dog ≥6.0 mg/dL, cat ≥5.5 mg/dL) occurs when the dynamic balance between osteosynthesis (calcium uptake) and osteolysis (calcium release) is altered, which causes excessive inhibition of sodium channels by excess calcium ions. Hypercalcemia also leads to reduced neuromuscular excitability, tissue irritation with deposition of calcium crystals, and stimulation of gastric secretory activity and contractile activity of the vascular muscle cells.

The causes of hypercalcemia are numerous:
- *Pseudohypercalcemia* due to increased calcium levels secondary to hyperproteinemia or hyperalbuminemia.
- *Nonsignificant hypercalcemia*, when hypercalcemia is considered normal in growing subjects or severely dehydrated patients.
- *Increased PTH production* due to primary hyperparathyroidism (parathyroid neoplasms) or secondary renal hyperparathyroidism.
- *Malignant neoplasms* such as T-cell lymphoma and various types of carcinomas (e.g., adenocarcinomas of the anal sacs) that stimulate excessive PTH production, monoclonal gammopathies responsible for an increase in calcium bound to paraproteins (such as multiple myeloma and some leukemias), and extensive bone metastases that cause bone lysis.
- *Increased absorption* of intestinal calcium due to an excessive intake (iatrogenic) or production of vitamin D, intoxications by some rodenticides and toxic plants, granulomatous diseases, and some neoplasms.
- *Reduced renal excretion* caused by acute or chronic kidney disease or by taking thiazide diuretics.
- *Corticosteroid deficiency* due to primary or secondary hypoadrenocorticism.
- Reduction of the proportion of calcium bound to proteins in *metabolic acidosis*.
- *Feline idiopathic hypercalcemia*, often associated with calcium oxalate urolithiasis, is diagnosed when no other cause is identified in this species. The origin is unknown, and affected cats have a low PTH value or at the lower limits of the norm [7–10].

Chapter 4 ◆ Electrolyte Disorders

Clinical signs

The most common signs of hypercalcemia are polyuria, polydipsia, anorexia, dehydration, lethargy, nausea, vomiting, and chronic kidney disease. Less common signs are constipation, arrhythmias, acute renal failure, calcium oxalate urolithiasis, muscle spasms, and convulsive states that, in the most severe forms, can lead to death. The rate at which hypercalcemia develops and its duration determine the severity of the clinical signs. In dogs, calcium values >15 mg/dL determine the onset of the first signs and values >20 mg/dL can be lethal.

Treatment

Patients are treated when calcium values are >16 mg/dL, or when values are lower but neurological or cardiac signs or alterations in renal function appear.

Once hypercalcemia has been diagnosed, it is necessary to first exclude all causes of artifacts before proceeding with one of the following treatments:
- Fluid therapy with 0.9% NaCl or another saline isotonic solution that does not contain calcium, especially if the patient is in metabolic acidosis. Fluid therapy must correct dehydration, if it is present, and produce a slight expansion of the circulating volume, so as to facilitate calciuresis. If fluid therapy is performed with saline, it should be supplemented with potassium chloride. The infusion rate of the solution should be about twice that used for maintenance fluids, taking special care not to cause tissue edema, especially in patients suffering from heart or kidney failure. In case of metabolic acidosis, sodium bicarbonate may be administered at a dose of 1 mEq/kg in a slow intravenous infusion.
- Administration of diuretics, such as furosemide at a dose of 2 mg/kg IV, SC, or orally every 8–12 hours, to promote calciuresis. Thiazide diuretics should not be used, as they involve hypocalciuria and aggravate hypercalcemia. When administering diuretics, it is essential to avoid dehydration and hypokalemia.
- Administration of glucocorticoids such as dexamethasone at a dose of 0.1–0.22 mg/kg/12 hours IV or SC, or prednisone at a dose of 1–2.2 mg/kg/12 hours IV, SC, or orally. These steroids have a dual action: they reduce bone resorption and calcium absorption in the intestine and increase its renal excretion. In addition, they help to treat the primary cause, such as lymphoma in cats, feline idiopathic hypercalcemia, anal sac adenocarcinoma, multiple myeloma, hypoadrenocorticism, hypervitaminosis D, and granulomatous pathologies.
- Administration of calcitonin at a dose of 4–6 IU/kg/8–12 hours SC for 24–48 hours. Hypervitaminosis D reduces the activity and formation of osteoclasts and the level of total calcium. Note that calcitonin can cause anorexia and vomiting and is very expensive.
- Administration of bisphosphonates (e.g., etidronate, pamidronate, clodronate) at a dose of 15 mg/kg/12–24 hours to reduce the activity of osteoclasts, by inducing

Chapter 4 ◆ Electrolyte Disorders

their apoptosis. They are also used to inhibit bone calcium resorption in the management of feline idiopathic hypercalcemia (see Box 4.3).

Phosphorus

Phosphorus is an essential mineral for bones, in which it is present in the form of hydroxyapatite. It is also contained in cells as a constituent of cAMP (cyclic adenosine monophosphate), ATP (adenosine triphosphate), NADP (nicotinamide adenine dinucleotide phosphate), phospholipids, and phosphoproteins (e.g., muscle phosphocreatine). A proportion of phosphorus is found in plasma as inorganic phosphate, as lipid phosphorus, and as an organic ester. Circulating phosphorus is measured by determining its inorganic form.

Most phosphorus (about 65–70%) is absorbed in the intestines, more particularly in the small intestine (duodenum and ileum) and to a lesser extent in the colon. The intestinal absorption process can be active, through a sodium-dependent cotransporter, or passive, by electrochemical gradient. The factors regulating the intestinal absorption of phosphorus are vitamin D, which enhances cotransporter function in the duodenum, and food deficiency, which activates renal hydroxylation of vitamin D to increase phosphorus absorption. Excessive oral doses of calcium cause a precipitation of phosphorus in the intestine. The remaining part is reabsorbed by the convoluted renal tubule, mainly the proximal convoluted tubule, thanks to the presence of a sodium-dependent active transport system. Factors that reduce tubular phosphorus absorption are the secretion of excessive amounts of PTH; a high amount of calcitonin, which increases renal excretion by increasing the filtered load; glucocorticoid intake, which hinders the sodium-dependent transport system by activating phosphorylation processes; and respiratory acidosis. The causes of an increase in the tubular absorption of phosphorus are the administration of insulin, which increases cellular phosphorus uptake for energy purposes and thus leads to a reduction in its urinary excretion; the administration of thyroid hormones, which are responsible for phosphorus retention; and respiratory alkalosis, which stimulates cellular phosphorus uptake due to hyperactivity of the respiratory muscles.

Hyperphosphatemia

Hyperphosphatemia (dog >7.4 mg/dL, cat >7.6 mg/dL) can be distinguished into significant and nonsignificant hyperphosphatemia. Insignificant increases in phosphorus can be due to analytical errors, i.e., the use of hyperlipidemic or hemolytic samples, and is a common finding in growing patients, in whom it is linked to the physiological processes of bone remodeling.

Significant increases in phosphorus, on the other hand, are due to several causes, which can be divided into the following categories:
- *Maldistribution of phosphorus*: lysis of cancer cells, rhabdomyolysis, tissue trauma, hemolysis and metabolic acidosis.
- *Increased intestinal absorption*: diets rich in phosphorus (in dogs), intake of laxatives containing phosphates, and hypervitaminosis D. The latter condition can be caused by excessive iatrogenic supplementation of vitamin D, intoxication with plants containing vitamin D, and poisoning with certain rodenticides.
- *Reduced renal excretion of phosphorus*: acute and chronic kidney disease, urethral obstruction, uroabdomen, hypoparathyroidism, and hyperthyroidism.

Clinical signs

Hyperphosphatemia causes hypocalcemia, which is responsible for the typical signs of reduced calcium concentration (e.g., muscle weakness, tetany, nausea, vomiting, arrhythmias; for more details see *Hypocalcemia*).

Treatment

Once hyperphosphatemia has been diagnosed, it is necessary to determine whether it is an increase due to analytical errors or a consequence of the conditions mentioned above. The patient's hydration status should then be assessed. In dehydrated patients, simple rehydration with an isotonic saline solution (e.g., 0.9% NaCl or Ringer's lactate) may be sufficient to reduce phosphorus through increased renal excretion. Therapy should also control intestinal absorption; the amount of phosphorus in the diet should be reduced by administering low-protein diets (low-protein foods are also low in phosphorus). In patients with acute or chronic kidney disease, phosphorus-chelating substances, such as aluminum hydroxide or aluminum carbonate, are administered to reduce intestinal absorption. The most widely used is aluminum hydroxide at a dose of 30 mg/kg/8 hours orally with meals, until phosphoremia is normalized. To correct hyperphosphatemia, it should not be forgotten that the most effective treatment is always to treat the cause (Box 4.4).

Hypophosphatemia

Hypophosphatemia is a pathological condition associated with reduced intestinal absorption of phosphorus due to anorexia, diets low in meat, intake of phosphorus binders such as aluminum hydroxide, malabsorption, or hypovitaminosis D, and with reduced renal reabsorption of phosphorus due to primary hyperparathyroidism, eclampsia, hyperadrenocorticism, or disorders of the proximal renal tubule (e.g., Fanconi syndrome).

Chapter 4 ◆ Electrolyte Disorders

Box 4.4	Treatment of phosphorus imbalances

Hyperphosphatemia: dog >7.4 mg/dL, cat >7.6 mg/dL

- Rehydration with 0.9% NaCl or Ringer's lactate solution.
- Low-protein diet.
- Aluminum hydroxide, 30 mg/kg/8 hours orally.

Hypophosphatemia: 1.0-2.0 mg/dL

- Potassium phosphate: 0.01–0.03 mmol/kg/hour IV in 0.9% NaCl or 5% glucose solution for 6 hours.
  Severe hypophosphatemia (<1 mg/dL): phosphate 0.03–0.12 mmol/kg/hour IV in 0.9% NaCl or 5% glucose solution.
- Typically, 2 hours of infusion every 6 hours is sufficient. Infuse up to 2 mg/dL blood. Usually, 2–4 treatments are enough.
- Dilute phosphate in calcium-free solutions.

Clinical signs

Hypophosphatemia leads to several alterations of blood cells, in particular erythrocytes, which may become more fragile due to a reduction in the concentration of ATP. This phenomenon may be responsible for intravascular hemolysis, especially when phosphorus is equal to or less than 1 mg/dL. Hypophosphatemia, in erythrocytes, is responsible for a reduction in the concentration of the enzyme 2,3-DPG, which decreases the ability of these cells to transport oxygen, resulting in poorer tissue oxygenation. Other consequences are thrombocytopenia and a reduction in chemotaxis and phagocytosis by leukocytes, with a greater predisposition to sepsis in patients at risk. Patients may show muscle weakness and pain associated with rhabdomyolysis, anorexia and vomiting secondary to paralytic ileus, and central nervous system disorders (e.g., irritability, confusional states and, in severe forms, coma).

Treatment

Only symptomatic patients are treated; treatment consists in the oral or parenteral administration of phosphorus. The oral route, using multivitamin and mineral preparations, is to be preferred over the parenteral route, as the intravenous administration of sodium phosphate or potassium phosphate (KH_2PO_4) can produce hyperphosphatemia with consequent hypocalcemia, renal failure, tetany, and mineralization phenomena. Potassium and sodium phosphate solutions contain 3 mmol of phosphate per milliliter and 4.4 mEq of potassium or 4 mEq of sodium per milliliter. The initial dose of phosphate is 0.01–0.03 mmol/kg/hour IV for 6 hours diluted in calcium-free

Chapter 4 ◆ Electrolyte Disorders

solutions (e.g., NaCl 0.9% or 5% glucose). In dogs and cats with severe hypophosphatemia, it may be necessary to increase the dosage from 0.03 to 0.12 mmol/kg/hour. Initially, it is important to monitor the serum phosphate concentration every 8–12 hours to correct supplementation. If the typical clinical signs of hypocalcemia appear during treatment, the rate of phosphate infusion should be decreased and ionized calcium, in addition to phosphorus, should also be monitored.

Chloride

Chloride is the main anion in the extracellular fluid and is essential in maintaining osmolarity and the acid–base balance. The normal serum chloride concentration is about 110–115 mEq/L in dogs and about 120–125 mEq/L in cats. The mechanisms of regulation of chloremia are closely linked to those of sodium, since much of the circulating chloride contributes, with bicarbonates, to maintaining electrolyte neutrality. It is therefore necessary to determine not only the patient's natremia but also their acid–base status to correctly interpret alterations in chloremia.

Alterations in chloremia accompanied by alterations in natremia in the same direction are caused by water balance problems (e.g., severe dehydration).

Alterations in chloremia that are not associated with equivalent changes in natremia are usually caused by acid–base imbalances. Chloride ions are constantly excreted in large amounts with gastric juices, and most of them are reabsorbed by the intestine. Chloride ions are filtered by concentration gradient across the glomeruli and reabsorbed by an active transport system in the ascending limb of the loop of Henle and in the distal portion of the proximal tubule of the nephron.

Hyperchloremia

Hyperchloremia may be due to preanalytical errors, such as dehydrated samples or samples from patients receiving potassium bromide.

Hyperchloremia is significant when associated with hypernatremia. In these cases, it can be produced by ECF imbalances, such as dehydration, or result from an increased intake or iatrogenic retention of chloride due to the administration of solutions containing high concentrations of NaCl, salt poisoning, hyperadrenocorticism, chronic respiratory alkalosis, renal failure, or diuretics (acetazolamide).

Iatrogenic hyperchloremia may be due to parenteral nutrition or to the administration of 0.9% NaCl and hypertonic solutions, potassium, or magnesium chloride. When associated with normo- or hyponatremia, it can be caused by acid–base imbalances (e.g., metabolic acidosis). Hypochloremia can be caused by diarrhea, vomiting,

Chapter 4 ◆ Electrolyte Disorders

renal loss of bicarbonate at the level of the proximal tubule, reduced renal excretion of H⁺ and chloride through the distal tubule, and chronic respiratory alkalosis. In the latter case, the kidney adapts to this chronic condition by increasing bicarbonate excretion and consequently reducing chloride excretion.

Clinical signs

Clinical signs of hyperchloremia are not pathognomonic. Some of them are attributable to the causes of metabolic acidosis.

Treatment

In cases of hyperchloremia it is necessary to determine the sodium-corrected chloride concentration, as shown in the following formula:

$$\text{Corrected Cl}^- = [Cl^-]_p \times [Na^+]_n / [Na^+]_p \qquad (Equation\ 9)$$

$[Cl^-]_p$, patient's blood chloride concentration; $[Na^+]_n$, normal blood sodium concentration; $[Na^+]_p$, patient's blood sodium concentration.
The normal value of [Na+] in dogs is 145 mEq/L, in cats it is 155 mEq/L.

If the corrected chloride value is normal, the patient should be rehydrated with intravenous fluids. If, however, the corrected chloride concentration is altered, metabolic acidosis must first be corrected by administering fluids (e.g., replenishment solution with sodium gluconate or Ringer's acetate) and, if necessary, sodium bicarbonate. The underlying cause that produced the acid–base disorder should also be treated for this electrolyte imbalance.

Hypochloremia

Hypochloremia is called pseudohypochloremia when the sample is severely lipemic or hyperproteinemic. True hypochloremia, on the other hand, can be associated with hyponatremia (the corrected chloride value is normal) and due to:
- loss of Cl⁻ and Na⁺ of renal, gastroenteric (e.g., vomiting) or cutaneous origin;
- sequestration of chloride and sodium in uroperitoneum and ascites;
- water retention in the course of congestive heart disease, cirrhotic liver disease, nephrotic syndrome and syndrome of inappropriate secretion of ADH (false hypochloremia);
- diuretics;
- transfer of water from ICF to ECF (e.g., in diabetes mellitus)
- chronic respiratory acidosis;
- hyperadrenocorticism.

Chapter 4 ♦ Electrolyte Disorders

Box 4.5	Treatment of chloride imbalances

Hyperchloremia
- Corrected Cl⁻ = $[Cl^-]_p \times [Na^+]_n/[Na^+]_p$
- If the corrected chloride concentration is normal, rehydrate the patient
- Correct acidosis with solutions with a high SID (e.g., Plasma-Lyte with sodium gluconate)

Hypochloremia
- Rehydratation with chloride-containing solutions (e.g., 0.9% NaCl or 0.45% solution)
- If the patient should not be administered more sodium, then potassium chloride, ammonium chloride, calcium chloride, or magnesium chloride can be used.

True hypochloremia may also be associated with normo- or hypernatremia (the corrected chloride value is decreased). This condition can be caused by metabolic alkalosis, since a reduction in chloride ions is associated with an increase in bicarbonate; by gastric torsion (gastric sequestration of HCl); and by administration of loop diuretics. True hypochloremia also occurs during metabolic acidosis (e.g., ketoacidosis, lactic acidosis, and ethylene glycol poisoning), since a reduction in chloremia is associated with a reduction in the concentration of bicarbonate. Chronic respiratory acidosis, which is responsible for a chronic increase in carbon dioxide, can induce hypochloremia by renal compensation of the respiratory acid–base imbalance (increased HCl secretion and HCO_3^- recovery).

Treatment

Treatment of hypochloremia involves correcting dehydration and the acid–base imbalance by providing fluid therapy appropriate to the patient's needs; it is therefore recommended to assess the patient's acid–base and electrolyte status prior to administering fluids. The underlying cause of hypochloremia must also be treated at the same time (Box 4.5).

Magnesium

Magnesium has received little attention in veterinary medicine and only several studies conducted in dogs and cats since 1970 have shown the importance of this electrolyte

Chapter 4 ◆ Electrolyte Disorders

in maintaining homeostasis and for cardiac and neuromuscular activity. The normal serum magnesium concentration in dogs is about 1.9–2.5 mg/dL. The exact distribution of magnesium in the body of animals is not yet fully understood; in humans, 99% of magnesium is found inside the cells and only 1% in the extracellular fluid. Approximately 67% is distributed in the bones, along with calcium and phosphorus, 20% in muscle tissue and 11% in other tissues. The remaining 1% in the extracellular fluid can be found in free form (55%), bound to proteins (20 to 30%), and in complex form (15 to 25%). The percentage of magnesium bound to proteins (especially albumins) is lower than that of calcium bound to proteins, so the concentration of magnesium is not very conditioned by changes in serum protein concentration. Most of the magnesium from the diet is absorbed by the ileum and a small part by the jejunum and colon. Magnesium is transported across the intestine by two mechanisms: a passive paracellular route and an active transcellular route. These different types of transport are also present in the kidney and their regulation depends on the concentration of calcium and some hormones, such as the parathyroid hormone. The kidney therefore plays a fundamental role in controlling and regulating the concentration of magnesium. Approximately about 10–15% of magnesium is filtered in the proximal tubule through passive transport, but this mechanism is not yet fully known; most magnesium (60–70%) is reabsorbed in the loop of Henle. Reabsorption is influenced by several factors: the positively charged luminal environment, which depends on the movements of sodium and chloride from the lumen to the interstitial space; sodium and water movements; the presence of special cation detection receptors (CASR, calcium-sensing receptors); and some hormones such as the parathyroid hormone, calcitonin, glucagon, antidiuretic hormone, aldosterone and insulin. These hormones promote the absorption of magnesium. Conversely, conditions of hypokalemia, hypophosphatemia, and metabolic acidosis reduce its absorption. As for the excretion of magnesium through urine, a fundamental role is played by the distal convoluted tubule, although the mechanisms by which it occurs are not fully understood. It seems that several hormones (see above), in certain conditions such as those mentioned above, and the presence of CASR and proteins such as TRMP6 and TRMP7 are responsible for the regulation of magnesium at the level of the distal convoluted tubule.

Hypomagnesemia

Etiology

The causes of hypomagnesemia are numerous and can be classified into three categories:
- gastrointestinal pathologies: chronic diarrhea, malnutrition, malabsorption syndrome, short bowel syndrome, intestinal neoplasm;

Chapter 4 ♦ Electrolyte Disorders

- renal pathologies: acute or chronic kidney disease, urethral obstruction, hyperaldosteronism and hyperthyroidism (which cause an increase in diuresis), renal tubular acidosis, and treatment with diuretics;
- various disorders: hyperglycemia, electrolytes disorders (hypokalemia, hypercalcemia, hyperparathyroidism, hypophosphatemia), diabetes mellitus, medications (e.g., gentamicin, cyclosporine, cisplatin), myocardial infarction, acute pancreatitis, excess catecholamines, excessive loss with lactation (especially in farm animals).

Diagnosis

The diagnosis of hypomagnesemia is complex since most of the magnesium is contained within the cells (99%). Its measurement may therefore not be reliable, as the measurement of its ion (Mg^{2+}) does not evaluate the total amount of magnesium present in the body. Its deficiency is often hypothesized based on the clinical presentation and the appearance of specific signs.

Clinical signs

Magnesium is fundamental in neuromuscular transmission and its deficiency leads to the appearance of muscle tetany and mental confusion (these clinical signs are rare in small animals, but more frequent in farm animals). It plays an important role in the contraction and excitability of striated muscles and in the contraction and conduction of the heart muscle.

This electrolyte is also fundamental in regulating the calcium concentration in muscle cells and the displacement of sodium and calcium within myocytes, as well as in regulating the concentration of potassium outside these cells. A magnesium deficiency can cause atrial fibrillation, supraventricular tachycardia, ventricular tachycardia, ventricular ectopic beats, and arrhythmias. Magnesium is also important for calcium regulation in the smooth muscles of the peripheral vascular system and its deficiency leads to vasoconstriction and, therefore, hypertension. Recent studies have shown the importance of magnesium in the production of inflammatory cytokines, such as tissue necrosis factor and interleukin 1. Typically, hypomagnesemia is associated with other electrolyte imbalances. The most frequent are hypokalemia and hypophosphatemia, with the characteristic clinical signs (see *Hypokalemia* and *Hypophosphatemia*). Refractory hypokalemia may be associated with hypomagnesemia; for this reason, in severe or non-treatment-responsive hypokalemia, magnesium measurement or supplementation during therapy is recommended.

Treatment

An adequate diet with specific dog or cat food is enough to prevent and treat states of hypomagnesemia. If magnesium deficiency is caused by gastrointestinal or kidney disease or the other conditions mentioned above, the causes should be treated.

Chapter 4 ♦ Electrolyte Disorders

The administration of magnesium in the form of magnesium sulfate or chloride, in dogs and cats, is empirical and no reliable data about this treatment are available. A possible therapy is the intravenous administration of magnesium sulfate or chloride at a dose of 0.2–0.3 mEq/kg and a rate of 0.12 mEq/kg/min, in 5% glucose solution for 24–48 hours. In severe forms of hypomagnesemia, 0.2–1.0 mEq/kg/day may be administered. During magnesium administration, the patient may experience vomiting, diarrhea, respiratory depression, weakness, hypotension, and cardiovascular collapse. Some electrolyte solutions contain magnesium; for example, Plasma-Lyte contains 3 mEq in 500 mL (see Table 3.1 in Chapter 3). Oral supplementation can be done with 1–2 mEq/kg/day (Box 4.6).

Hypermagnesemia

States of hypermagnesemia are rare in veterinary medicine and very few studies are available about this imbalance. Two significant studies have been conducted so far. In the first one, 11 cats treated with methylprednisolone acetate following dermatitis experienced an increase in magnesium after 3–6 days, but it was not considered clinically significant [11]. In the other study, 50 small dogs with mitral valve insufficiency were treated with spironolactone and an angiotensin inhibitor, and an increase in magnesium levels was observed after 20 days, but again this was not considered clinically significant [12]. Forms with severe clinical signs, such as arrhythmias, unconsciousness, respiratory depression, and risk of death, can be treated with 10% calcium gluconate at a dose of 0.5–1.5 mg/kg IV in a slow infusion (over 10–15 minutes), as calcium gluconate acts as an antagonist at the neuromuscular junction, or with physostigmine at a dose of 0.02 mg/kg/12 hours IV (see Box 4.6).

Box 4.6 — **Treatment of magnesium imbalances**

Hypomagnesemia: <1.5 mg/dL
- Magnesium sulfate or chloride 0.2–0.3 mEq/kg, at 0.12 mEq/kg/min, diluted up to <20% in 0.9% NaCl or 5% glucose.
- Do not use solutions containing lactate and calcium bicarbonate.
- Severe hypomagnesemia: 0.2–1.0 mEq/kg/day.
- Oral supplementation: 1–2 mEq/kg/day.

Hypermagnesemia
- Symptomatic therapy.
- Severe: 10% calcium gluconate 0.5–1.5 mg/kg IV in slow infusion or physostigmine 0.02 mg/kg/12 hours IV.

Chapter 4 ◆ Electrolyte Disorders

References

[1] DiBartola SP. *Fluid, Electrolyte, and Acid-Base Disorders in Small Animal Practice*, 4th ed. St. Louis: Elsevier Saunders; 2012.

[2] Brofman PJ, Knostman KA, DiBartola SP. Granulomatous amebic meningoencephalitis causing the syndrome of inappropriate secretion of antidiuretic hormone in a dog. *J Vet Intern Med*. 2003;17(2):230–234.

[3] Moritz ML, Ayus JC. Hospital-acquired hyponatremia: why are hypotonic parenteral fluids still being used? *Nat Clin Pract Nephrol*. 2007;3(7):374–382.

[4] Peterson ME, Kintzer PP, Kass PH. Pretreatment clinical and laboratory findings in dogs with hypoadrenocorticism: 225 cases (1979-1993). *J Am Vet Med Assoc*. 1996;208(1):85–91.

[5] O'Brien DP, Kroll RA, Johnson GC et al. Myelinolysis after correction of hyponatremia in two dogs. *J Vet Intern Med*. 1994;8(1):40–48.

[6] Lind L, Carlstedt F, Rastad J et al. Hypocalcemia and parathyroid hormone secretion in critically ill patients. *Crit Care Med*. 2000;28(1):93–99.

[7] [Paltrinieri S, Bertazzolo W, Giordano A. *Clinical Pathology of Dogs and Cats: Practical Approach to Laboratory Diagnostics*. Milan: Elsevier; 2010.

[8] Harvey A, Tasker S. *BSAVA. Manuale di Medicina Felina*. Milan: Edra; 2014.

[9] Viganò F. *Manuale di pronto soccorso nel cane e nel gatto*. Milan: Edra; 2013.

[10] Thompson MS. *Small Animal Medical Differential Diagnosis*, 2nd ed. St. Louis: Elsevier Saunders; 2014.

[11] Sharkey LC, Ployngam T, Tobias AH et al. Effects of a single injection of methylprednisolone acetate on serum biochemical parameters in 11 cats. *Vet Clin Pathol*. 2007;36:184.

[12] Thomason JD, Rockwell JE, Fallaw TK et al. Influence of combined angiotensin-converting enzyme inhibitors and spironolactone on serum K^+, Mg^{2+}, and Na^+ concentration in small dog with degenerative mitral valve disease. *J Vet Cardiol*. 2007;9(2):103–108.

Clinical Case

Electrolyte and acid–base imbalances during vomiting

Prevalence				
Technical difficulty				

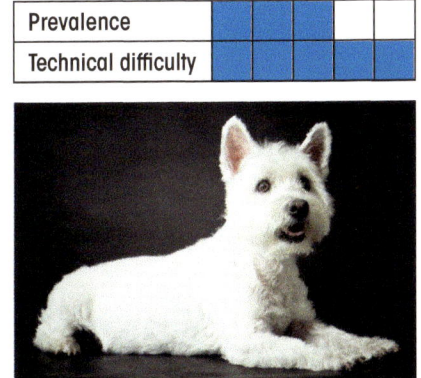

Signalment	
Name	Snow
Species	canine
Breed	West Highland White Terrier
Sex	male
Weight	5 kg
Age	1 year

History

The patient was brought to the clinic because he had not been eating since the previous day and had experienced about 10 episodes of vomiting per day for the previous 2 days. His last stools (the previous day) were normal in consistency, but mucus was present on their surface.

At triage, the patient's following vital parameters were as follows:
- heart rate: 150 bpm;
- respiratory rate: 23 bpm;
- full pulse;
- rectal temperature: 38.1 °C;
- mucous membranes: pink, CRT 1.5 seconds;
- blood pressure: 145/113 mmHg; MAP: 124 mmHg;
- 10% dehydration.

Laboratory tests

A blood gas analysis was performed because the patient had vomited numerous times and, given its young age, he was at risk of severe electrolyte and acid-base

Chapter 4 ♦ Electrolyte Disorders

imbalances. In these cases, a blood gas analysis is useful to provide fluids that meet the patient's requirements and can correct any electrolyte and acid-base or disorders. A blood count was performed to check for any hematological alterations, especially in the hematocrit and leukocytes. A biochemistry profile was also used to detect possible dysfunctions in the organs related to the digestive system and to identify, with the nontraditional approach to acid-base balance, any other potential metabolic components.

Venous blood gas analysis

Given that there was no problem with the respiratory system, a venous blood sample was taken, since the values obtained with this type of blood sample are reliable with regard to pH, bicarbonate and carbon dioxide levels, and, more especially in this case, electrolytes. The first blood gas analysis yielded the following results:
- pH 7.65;
- $pvCO_2$ 55;
- HCO_3^- 45;
- BE +35;
- Na^+ 125 mmol/L;
- Cl^- 84 mmol/L;
- K^+ 2.4 mmol/L;
- lactate 4.8 mmol/L;
- AG 2.4;
- FiO_2 0.21.

Biochemistry profile

BUN 45 mg/dL, creatinine 0.8 mg/dL, ALT 12 U/L, AST 27 U/L, total proteins 8.1 g/dL, albumin 3.5 g/dL, Bilirubin Tot 0.1 mg/dL, GGT 9 U/L, blood glucose 112 mg/100 mL, phosphorus 3.1 mg/dL.

Blood count

RBC 4.5×10^{12}/L, WBC 12.1×10^9/L, Hct 65%, Hb 22 g/dL, PLT 439×10^9/L, neutrophils 10×10^3/µL.

Interpretation of laboratory tests

The traditional approach to blood gas analysis highlighted a severe metabolic alkalosis because bicarbonate was significantly increased (45) and carbon dioxide was increased (respiratory acidosis) as a result of compensation. It was therefore a case of simple metabolic alkalosis with respiratory compensation, but with severe sodium, chloride and potassium imbalances. Lactic acidosis was also present, which was unlikely to be of circulatory origin, as the hemodynamic parameters detected did not point to a circulatory failure, but rather to a gastric wall lesion. According to the nontraditional approach, severe metabolic alkalosis and SID reduction alkalosis (-8 nmol/L) were present. There was a noticeable increase in unmeasured cations. In this case, there was no reason to suspect an increase in sulfates, so increases in calcium and magnesium or the presence of paraproteinemia were suspected. The A_{tot} did not compensate for alkalosis like respiratory acidosis.

Severe hyponatremia and hypochloremia were present and needed to be treated. The biochemistry profile highlighted an increase in proteinemia due to dehydration. The blood count showed an increased hematocrit, probably due to dehydration. The calculation of blood osmolarity was therefore carried out as follows:

$$Osm = 2 \times [Na^+] + glucose\ (mg/dL)/18 + BUN\ (mg/dL)/2.8$$

$$Osm = (2 \times 125) + (112/18) + (45/2.8)$$

$$Osm = 272\ mOsm/L$$

Osmolarity was lower than normal as a result of severe hyponatremia.

Chapter 4 ◆ Electrolyte Disorders

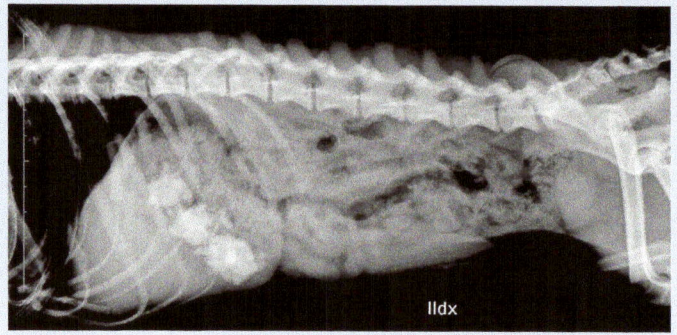

Diagnostic investigations

An X-ray of the abdomen was taken and revealed the presence of gastric foreign bodies of an unidentified nature.

Daily fluid therapy

Since the hemodynamic parameters were normal and there were no signs of hypovolemic shock, it was decided to provide maintenance fluid therapy, to which a volume of fluids corresponding to the percentage of dehydration (10%) was added.
Maintenance fluid therapy: 2 mL/kg/hour IV, which corresponds to 10 mL/hour.
Rehydration: 10% of 5 kg corresponds to 500 mL which, divided by 24 hours, corresponds to about 21 mL/hour IV.
So, the total amount of fluids to be infused per hour for at least 24 hours was 31 mL/hour IV.
In this case, since there was dehydration with severe hyponatremia, the volume of solution to be infused was calculated based on the measured sodium concentration. It was decided to infuse 0.9% NaCl to quickly restore both sodium and chloride losses. The calculation was made using the following equation:

$$(140 - [Na^+]_p) \times kg \times 0.3 = Na^+ \text{ deficit}$$

$$(140 - 125) \times 5 \times 0.3 = 22.5 \text{ mEq/L (patient's sodium deficit)}$$

Clinical Case

The sodium deficit was then divided by the sodium concentration of the solution used. In this case, 0.9% NaCl solution contains 154 mEq/L of sodium, so the volume in liters to be administered was calculated with the following formula:

$$Na^+ \text{ deficit}/[Na^+] \text{ of the solution} = \text{volume in liters of solution to be administered}$$

$$22.5/154 = 0.15 \text{ L}$$

To calculate the duration of administration, the following formula can be used:

$$(140 - [Na^+]_p)/0.5 = \text{number of hours of fluid therapy}$$

$$(140 - 125)/0.5 = 30 \text{ hours}$$

The initial administration rate calculated for the first 24 hours (31 mL/hour) meant that 744 mL of fluids would be administered in 24 hours, so it was decided to slow down the rate of administration to about half (15 mL/hour) of what had initially been calculated and then to repeat the blood gas analysis to monitor the correction obtained. The calculated volume of fluids was enough to restore sodium losses. It was decided not to further reduce the infusion rate due to the patient's severe dehydration. NaCl 0.9% solution is preferable to restore sodium and, because it has a zero SID and contains large amounts of chloride, it is also useful for correcting metabolic alkalosis. Potassium must be added to the solution using the table for its replenishment (see Table 4.1), which indicates 30 mEq/L of potassium chloride in 500 mL of isotonic saline solution. To correctly infuse the solution, it is necessary to use an infusion pump; the acid–base status should be monitored at least after 24 hours and the patient's weight should be monitored twice a day.

After 24 hours, the venous blood gas analysis was repeated and revealed the following results:
- pH 7.42;
- $pvCO_2$ 42;
- HCO_3^- 28;
- BE +2;
- Na^+ 135 mmol/L;
- Cl^- 110 mmol/L;

Chapter 4 ◆ Electrolyte Disorders

- K+ 3.5 mmol/L;
- lactate 2.0 mmol/L;
- AG 0.5;
- FiO2 0.21.

The patient underwent a gastroscopy, which enabled the removal of three ingested plastic foreign bodies (see figure below). On the second day, dehydration was reduced to about 8%, so the rate of fluid therapy was reduced according to the following calculation:

Maintenance fluid therapy: 2 mL/kg/hour IV, which corresponds to 10 mL/hour.

Rehydration: 8% of 5 kg corresponds to 400 mL which, divided by 24 hours, corresponds to about 17 mL/hour IV. The administration rate was therefore kept at 15 mL/hour on day 2. On day 3, the patient received only maintenance fluid therapy at 10 mL/hour IV.

The dog was discharged on day 3, once hydration had been restored and he had resumed feeding and drinking spontaneously.

Home supportive care involved a proton pump inhibitor for about 7 days (pantoprazole 1 mg/kg every 12 hours orally) and an intestinal adsorbent (diosmectite 1 g every 8 hours orally for 7 days) to facilitate healing of the necrotic ulcerative lesions found during the gastroscopy.

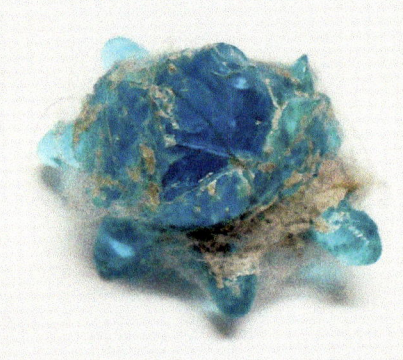

Clinical Case

Hemorrhagic shock following a ruptured hepatocellular carcinoma

Prevalence					
Technical difficulty					

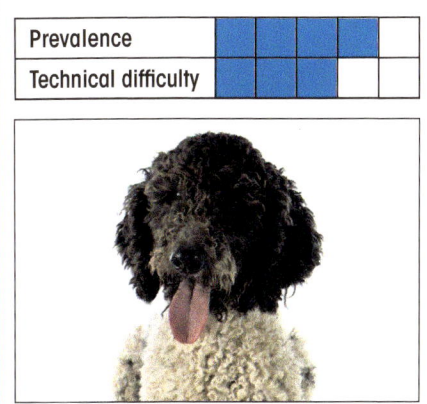

Signalment	
Name	Chloe
Species	canine
Breed	Portuguese Water Dog
Sex	female
Weight	25 kg
Age	8 years

An 8-year-old spayed female Portuguese Water Dog weighing 25 kg was presented to the emergency room after collapsing during a walk. She had a 3-day history of waxing and waning lethargy and a decreased appetite. There was no history of trauma, toxin ingestion, or relevant previous medical history.

On presentation, she was mentally obtunded with pale mucous membranes, weak femoral pulses, absent dorsal pedal pulses, a capillary refill time of 3 seconds, and cool extremities. Her rectal temperature was 35.3 °C, her heart rate 180 bpm, and her respiratory rate 60 bpm. She had no external evidence of wounds. Cardiothoracic auscultation revealed no murmurs or irregular rhythms and no crackles or wheezes, but she was taking short, shallow breaths. Her abdomen was distended with a palpable fluid wave and apparent pain on cranial abdominal palpation. Her Doppler blood pressure was 50 mmHg.

This patient was in the early stages of decompensatory shock with a concern for hemorrhagic shock due to a suspected fluid-filled abdomen. There were classic signs of shock and baroreceptor-mediated reflexes (vasoconstriction and tachycardia), but the Doppler blood pressure remained dangerously low. The compensatory mechanisms were not enough to improve perfusion to vital organs. Late decompen-

Chapter 5 ♦ Hemorrhagic Shock

satory shock is characterized by vasodilation and bradycardia due to sympathoinhibition; urgent intervention is needed to prevent progression to this irreversible state. An 18 gauge, 0.75" intravenous catheter was placed in her right cephalic vein. The patient was given a 500 mL (20 mL/kg) bolus of PlasmaLyte. An AFAST examination showed a large volume of free fluid in all four quadrants. A peripheral venous blood gas showed the following results:

- pH: 6.942;
- pCO_2: 53.6 mmHg;
- pO_2: 25.8 mmHg;
- Na: 139.5 mmol/L;
- K: 3.76 mmol/L;
- Cl: 110.2 mmol/L;
- Glu: 26 mmol/L;
- Lactate: 9.6 mmol/L;
- BE: -20.8 mmol/L;
- HCO_3^-: 11.7 mmol/L;
- PCV; 34%;
- TP; 4.2 g/dL.

These results indicate a marked lactic acidosis consistent with the poor perfusion and anaerobic metabolism seen in shock. The patient's hypercapnia without compensation could be due to her abnormal mentation caused by cerebral ischemia. Her hyperglycemia was likely due to increased sympathetic tone. Her PCV was likely higher than expected secondary to splenic contraction, with a low TP due to fluid shifting from the interstitial and subendothelial glycocalyx compartments.

An abdominocentesis was performed, and the effusion appeared bloody with a PCV of 36% and TP of 6.2 g/dL. This similarity between the peritoneal effusion PCV and peripheral PCV raised concern for active bleeding into the peritoneal cavity. After the initial PlasmaLyte bolus, the patient remained dull; her Doppler blood pressure was 60 mmHg and her heart rate was 170 bpm. She was given another 500 mL bolus of PlasmaLyte; her Doppler blood pressure remained at 60 mmHg and her heart rate improved to 160 bpm. Her PCV had decreased to 25% with a TP of 3.9 g/dL. A DEA 1.2(-) blood type was obtained, and she was given 300 mL (12 mL/kg) of pRBCs over 30 minutes. Her heart rate remained at 160 bpm, but her blood pressure

Clinical Case

improved to 80 mmHg. She appeared clinically brighter and had a better pulse quality. A repeat venous blood gas showed the following results:
- pH: 7.077;
- pCO_2: 47.6 mmHg;
- pO_2: 38.7 mmHg;
- Na: 140.4 mmol/L;
- K: 3.33 mmol/L;
- Cl: 115.6 mmol/L;
- Glu: 10.6 mmol/L;
- Lactate: 6.7 mmol/L;
- BE: -14.1 mmol/L;
- $HCO3^-$: 14.1 mmol/L;
- PCV: 35%;
- TP: 3.8 g/dL.

Following pRBC transfusion, the patient's PCV had appropriately increased, but her TP remained low. Her lactate level had slightly improved, along with her blood glucose and pCO_2. Her pO_2, although it was collected from a peripheral vein and was therefore not indicative of arterial or mixed venous oxygenation, had also improved, indicating improved tissue oxygenation following pRBC administration.

PT/PTT were normal. She was given 250 mL (10 mL/kg) FFP over 30 minutes. Her blood pressure rose to 90 mmHg and her pulse quality continued to improve. An abdominal ultrasound was performed and showed a large, cavitated mass associated with the left medial liver lobe and a large amount of free fluid. Thoracic radiographs showed no evidence of metastasis. A full chemistry showed her albumin was 1.2 g/dL. She was then administered a transfusion of 6 grams of canine albumin targeting a desired albumin of 2.0 g/dL (albumin dose = [desired albumin – patient albumin] × 25 kg × 0.3).

Following albumin transfusion, the patient's Doppler blood pressure was 140 mmHg and her heart rate improved to 107 beats per minute. Now hemodynamically stable, she was prepared for general anesthesia and surgery. Just prior to general anesthesia, a final venous blood gas showed:
- pH: 7.301;
- pCO_2: 40.2 mmHg;

Chapter 5 ♦ Hemorrhagic Shock

- pO_2: 35.2 mmHg;
- Na: 145.8 mmol/L;
- K: 3.51 mmol/L;
- Cl: 114.2 mmol/L;
- Glu: 5.1 mg/dL;
- Lactate: 2.3 mmol/L;
- BE: -4.6 mmol/L;
- $HCO3^-$: 20.0 mmol/L;
- PCV: 30%;
- TP: 4.4 g/dL.

Following FFP and albumin administration, her TS improved, but her PCV worsened following initial improvement after pRBC transfusion. Since she was likely continuing to bleed into her abdomen, damage control surgery was recommended to control the hemorrhage as quickly as possible. Despite this ongoing bleeding, adequate resuscitation led to an improved metabolic acidosis, lactate, pCO_2 and pO_2, thus optimizing her chances of successful surgery.

A laparotomy was performed, and a large volume of hemorrhagic effusion was present within the peritoneal cavity. A total of 400 mL of blood was collected from the abdomen into a sterile fluid bag. Anticoagulant (56 mL of citrate phosphate dextrose adenine) was added to the collected blood (0.14 mL anticoagulant per mL of blood) before IV administration as an autotransfusion.

During surgery, the left medial liver lobe, which contained a large, actively bleeding mass was isolated and removed. The dog recovered well from surgery and histopathology was consistent with a hepatocellular carcinoma.

While the most common cause for a neoplastic hemoabdomen is a malignant hemangiosarcoma, a massive ruptured hepatocellular carcinoma can carry a good prognosis. Proper stabilization and resuscitation are key to a successful outcome, particularly when the patient is presented in hemorrhagic shock.

The Microcirculation and Fluid Therapy

Deborah C. Silverstein

Introduction

When assessing and monitoring unstable animals, both objective and subjective indicators of tissue perfusion are often used to determine the amount and rate of fluid to be administered, if indicated. These indicators include parameters such as mentation, mucous membrane color, capillary refill time, pulse quality, extremity temperature, heart rate, and blood pressure (see Chapter 3). Although these are valid markers of macrovascular blood flow, they are unable to assess the smaller vessels and capillary beds, where gas and nutrient exchange occurs, also known as the microcirculation. Unfortunately, clinical evaluation of the microcirculation is not easily performed, and clinicians must therefore rely on global markers of macrocirculatory perfusion when evaluating sick animals. However, there are many diseases in which microcirculatory hypoperfusion is present despite normal macrocirculatory parameters (also known as cryptic shock or hemodynamic incoherence). This chapter will review the structure, function, and regulation of the microcirculation, changes that occur with disease states, and current methods for assessment. A clinical case illustrating the importance of microcirculatory perfusion is also presented.

Structure and function of the microcirculation

The microcirculatory unit is comprised of arterioles that feed into a capillary bed and are drained by venules (Figure 6.1). Precapillary arterioles have smooth muscle throughout, but terminal metarterioles have interrupted bands of smooth muscle. The walls of true capillaries contain no muscle and consist of one layer of endothelial cells attached to a basement membrane. Arterioles and venules are less than 100 µm in diameter, while capillaries are less than 10 µm in diameter [1]. Specialized shunt vessels allow arterial blood to bypass the associated microcirculatory unit, as dictated by arteriolar and precapillary sphincter tone [1]. The vascular endothelial surface layer (ESL) is present on the intimal surface of blood vessels and contains the endothelial glycocalyx and associated components from the endothelial cells

Chapter 6 ◆ The Microcirculation and Fluid Therapy

and plasma [2–3]. The ESL is between 200 nm and 2 μm thick and makes up about 25% of the vascular space [4]. The glycocalyx is comprised of a negatively charged carbohydrate rich gel-like layer that creates a barrier between the vessel wall and the blood [5–7]. It contains membrane-bound proteoglycans, secreted glycosaminoglycans, sialic acid–containing glycoproteins, and glycolipids that are associated with the vascular endothelial surface [8]. Proteins such as albumin and antithrombin are also contained within the glycocalyx [8–10]. The ESL functions to maintain the vascular permeability barrier; modulate nitric oxide (NO) production in response to shear stress; retain protective enzymes such as superoxide dismutase; inhibit coagulation via factors such as antithrombin, tissue factor pathway inhibitor, and protein C; assist with mechanotransduction; and prevent leukocyte adhesion and binding of ligands to control local inflammation [3,11]. Based on recent research examining the ESL, the Starling principle of transvascular fluid flux has been revised to include the oncotic pressure gradient between the plasma and glycocalyx rather than between the plasma and interstitial space (see Chapter 1) [12].

The microcirculation is the largest vascular surface area in the body and is vital for effective delivery of oxygen and nutrients to the cells and removal of waste products from tissue beds [1]. Both systemic and local regulation of blood flow through these units and maintenance of the ESL are essential to maintain adequate perfusion and match metabolic demand to oxygen/nutrient delivery.

Microvascular perfusion – systemic control

Vascular tone depends on many endogenous chemical mediators, such as catecholamines, endothelin and thromboxane (Box 6.1). Catecholamines are released in response to baro- or chemoreceptor activation of the sympathetic nervous system [13]. Baroreceptors respond to changes in blood pressure (stretching of the vessel wall) and chemoreceptors respond to chemical changes in the blood such as hypoxia, hypercapnia, or acidemia. Their effects are most critical when the systemic arterial pressure falls below 80 mmHg and catecholamines help to maintain perfusion in individual capillary beds despite a decreased systemic blood pressure [13].

However, true capillaries do not have sympathetic innervation or smooth muscle like the arteries and most of the venous vessels. Therefore, blood flow through each capillary bed is regulated by the hemodynamic pressures generated between the precapillary sphincter and the postcapillary venules. Since each capillary bed may be supplied by multiple arterioles, flow through the capillary bed can increase by 200–500% without any significant change in the arteriolar pressure [14]. This mechanism helps to preserve microcirculatory flow to specific tissue beds during periods of transient systemic hypotension in healthy animals.

Chapter 6 ◆ The Microcirculation and Fluid Therapy

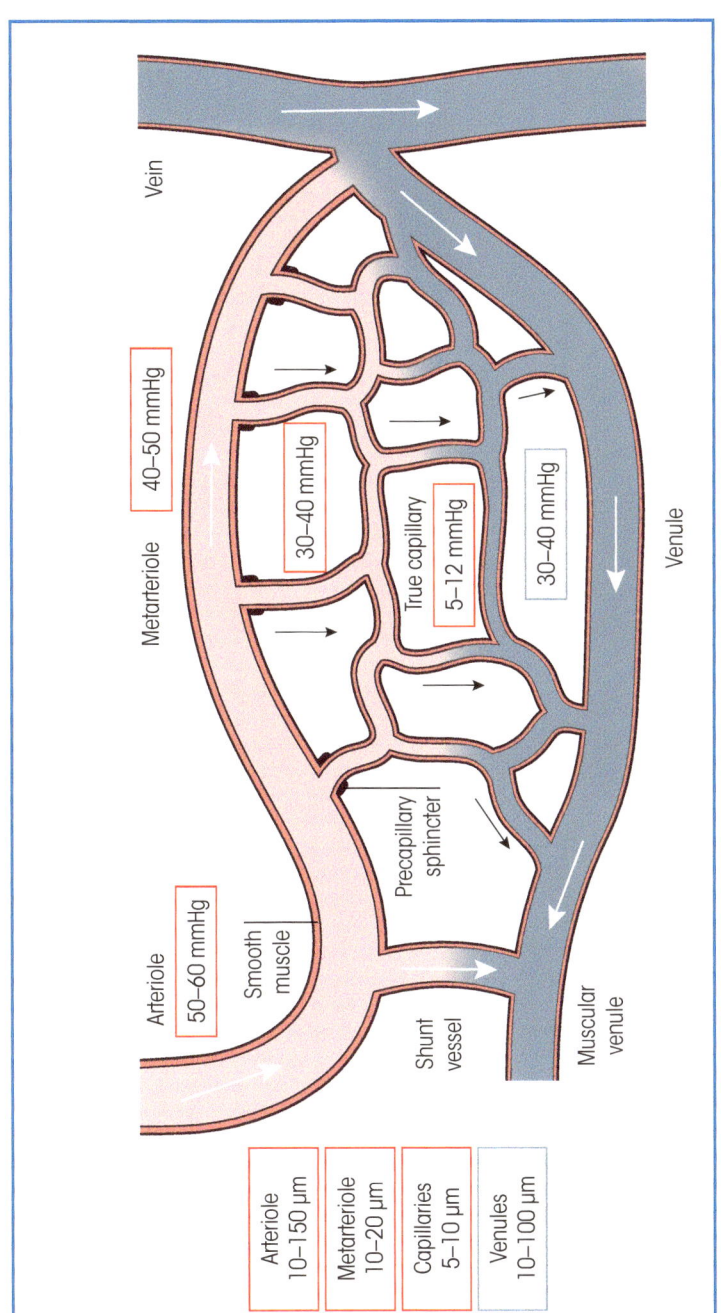

Figure 6.1 Schematic of the microcirculation. Boxes on the left represent ranges of vessel diameters at varying levels of the microcirculation. Boxes throughout the diagram represent the average interstitial (tissue) oxygen tension (P_tO_2). The arrows represent the direction of blood flow across the microcirculatory unit. From: Cooper ES, Silverstein DC. Fluid Therapy and the Microcirculation in Health and Critical Illness. *Front Vet Sci.* 2021;8:625708. doi: 10.3389/fvets.2021.625708

Chapter 6 ♦ The Microcirculation and Fluid Therapy

Box 6.1	Endogenous mediators of vascular smooth muscle tone
Vasoconstrictors: • Angiotensin II • Alkalosis • Endothelin • Endothelium-derived constricting factor • Epinephrine/norepinephrine • Hypothermia • Hyperoxia • Thromboxane A2 • Vasopressin	**Vasodilators:** • Acidosis • Carbon dioxide • Endothelium-derived hyperpolarizing factor • Histamine • Hyperthermia • Hypoxia • Increased tissue potassium, ADP, or adenosine • Kinins • NO • Prostacyclin

In addition to vascular tone, intravascular volume is also important for the maintenance of systemic blood pressure and tissue perfusion. The renin–angiotensin–aldosterone system plays a major role in the maintenance of adequate blood volume via sodium and water retention in the kidneys, and in increasing vascular smooth muscle tone via angiotensin II–mediated vasoconstriction [4,15]. Stimulation of vasopressin release causes further retention of free water and can influence vasomotor tone in certain situations [15].

Endogenous vasodilators are also important for increasing flow to capillary beds; these include kinins (bradykinin and l-lysl-bradykinin), adrenomedullin and atrial natriuretic peptide (ANP). They frequently work to regulate local blood flow but may also enter the systemic circulation. Bradykinin also increases capillary permeability, thereby augmenting nutrient delivery to the tissue bed [16]. Similarly, histamine acts to cause vasodilation and increased capillary permeability when released in response to tissue damage or allergic reactions. Adrenomedullin exerts its vasodilatory action by increasing the production of NO while ANP antagonizes various vasoconstrictor agents [16].

These chemical regulators are responsible for controlling the delivery of blood to precapillary sphincters across the different tissue beds throughout the cardiovascular system. Once blood arrives at a capillary bed, local regulatory mechanisms act to maintain flow through this capillary bed. This may function independent of systemic changes to perfusion [16].

Chapter 6 ◆ The Microcirculation and Fluid Therapy

Microvascular perfusion – local control

Each capillary bed has local regulators of microcirculatory flow that adjust perfusion based on local tissue metabolic rate, nutrient availability, and accumulation of waste products (Box 6.1). This causes precapillary sphincters to open or close (microcirculatory shunting) according to an increase or decrease in blood flow requirements, respectively. Adjustments in capillary perfusion are vital for modulating cardiac workload based on individual tissue bed demands [16].

Rapid mechanisms for the control of microcirculatory flow are mediated at a local level via autoregulation. For example, flow autoregulation using vascular stretch receptors maintains consistent capillary blood flow over a wide range of arterial pressures. An increase in systemic vascular pressure leads to increased tone of the precapillary sphincter, which mutes transmission of the pressure through the capillary circuit [17]. The opposite occurs when there is a decrease in peripheral pressure. This mechanism is independent of any neurohormonal input and can maintain consistent blood flow when the mean arterial pressure is 60–160 mmHg.

Variations in the metabolic demand of local tissues can greatly impact the control of blood flow to associated capillary beds. An increase in metabolic activity produces carbon dioxide, lactate, and hydrogen ions, which stimulate vasodilation to enhance local blood flow and increase oxygen/nutrient delivery. Even though these metabolites flow downstream, the countercurrent flow between arterioles and venules allows them to be "sensed" at the level of the precapillary sphincter, with a subsequent increase in blood flow [17]. Additionally, intercell and local neural pathways respond by enabling conduction of signals from the capillary endothelium and venular smooth muscle [17].

Microcirculatory regulation also depends on the local oxygen tension (PO_2). Normally, capillary blood has a significantly lower PO_2 (5–12 mmHg) than arteriolar blood (~60 mmHg) due to three mechanisms: early off-loading of oxygen in precapillary tissues, endothelial oxygen consumption, and countercurrent exchange with venous blood [17]. An increase in precapillary tissue PO_2 stimulates vasoconstriction, whereas a decrease results in vasodilation, largely through the release of NO. The role of NO in the regulation of microvascular tone is important in health and disease [17]. In healthy animals, the constitutive form of NO synthetase (cNOS) is responsible for maintaining a basal level of NO to modulate vascular tone and meet tissue demands. In disease states that cause blood hyperviscosity, such as polycythemia vera or severe hemoconcentration, the increase in vascular endothelial shear stress leads to an increase in cNOS, an increase in NO, and subsequent vasodilation. In contrast, patients with severe anemia/hemodilution and a marked reduction in red cell mass have decreased blood viscosity and less of a stimulus for vasodilation [18]. The inducible form of NO synthetase (iNOS) can be produced by the endothelial cells when triggered by inflammation and cytokines. Prostacyclin-induced vasodilation may be important for producing a normal response to hypoxia, especially when NO is inhibited [19].

Chapter 6 ◆ The Microcirculation and Fluid Therapy

Microvascular changes with trauma and hemorrhagic shock

Patients suffering from trauma, acute pain, or hemorrhage experience rapid stimulation of the sympathetic nervous system and subsequent release of epinephrine and norepinephrine; this leads to vasoconstriction, particularly in the large arterioles (70–150 μm) that supply skeletal muscles [20]. The response is variable in the smaller arterioles (10–25 μm) with constriction in some capillary beds and dilation in others, mostly dictated by metabolic demand and the relative hierarchy of vital organs (e.g., the brain and heart are a priority).

The tone of the small arterioles will decrease (i.e., small arterioles will dilate) following trauma and hemorrhage resulting in decreased tissue oxygen delivery. However, this change is counteracted by inhibition of endothelial NO synthase (eNOS) in the early stages following trauma and hemorrhage. As iNOS is upregulated secondary to tissue damage and cytokine release, there is an increase in vasodilation [21]. An assortment of vasoactive mediators with mixed effects will also be released and a progressive acidosis and accumulation of cellular metabolites (particularly in the terminal stages of shock) will then further promote vasodilation and reverse systemic vasoconstrictive efforts. This can result in a decrease in driving pressure in the face of hypotension that ultimately leads to stagnation of blood flow.

The venous circulation also plays a role in the maintenance of microvascular perfusion. Immediately following trauma and hemorrhage, catecholamine-induced venoconstriction acts to decrease venous capacitance and increase the return of blood to the heart. As shock progresses, however, a more diffuse relaxation (through mechanisms similar to those described above) causes pooling of blood in the venous circulation, which may lead to downstream stagnation of blood flow with negative implications on capillary perfusion and oxygen delivery.

Several additional factors may contribute to abnormal microcirculatory flow. Patients with systemic inflammation, shock, or trauma may have vascular endothelial cell swelling due to increased membrane permeability, acidosis, and impaired electrolyte transport from failure of ATP-dependent channels [22]. A decrease in the capillary lumen from endothelial swelling can adversely affect capillary blood flow and patency. In addition, endothelial cell edema may also impair the release of prostacyclin and NO while increasing that of endothelin and thromboxane; the net effect is upstream vasoconstriction, which further compromises capillary flow. Oxidative injury, ATP deficiencies, cell membrane injury, and cellular dehydration may also decrease red blood cell (RBC) deformability through the narrow capillaries [22]. In normal patients, RBCs are slightly larger than the capillary lumen; therefore, their folding is necessary to flow through the microcirculation. The inability to fold, along

Chapter 6 ◆ The Microcirculation and Fluid Therapy

with aggregation, may result in capillary plugging and/or shearing injury/premature destruction of RBCs. Additionally, increased rigidity and endothelial adherence of leukocytes may lead to arteriolar and capillary plugging. Finally, the microthrombi that form because of tissue/endothelial injury, the inflammatory response, and hypercoagulability may become lodged at various levels of the microcirculation and impede downstream flow.

The deleterious upstream and downstream effects have the potential to greatly impact capillary flow and delivery of oxygen and nutrients to tissues. Vasoconstriction leads to shunting of blood away from the capillary bed (decreased vessel numbers), while hypotension, vasodilation, and obstruction leads to stagnation of blood (decreased flow). These derangements may persist for a prolonged time following resuscitation, despite normalization of macrovascular parameters [22–23].

Shedding of the endothelial glycocalyx has been seen in experimental rodent models of nontraumatic hemorrhagic shock, although the changes are independent of increased vascular endothelial permeability [24–26].

Microvascular changes with sepsis

The progression of untreated sepsis leads to systemic deterioration and culminates in septic shock, a condition originally defined as the presence of refractory hypotension, hyperlactatemia, and organ dysfunction that persists despite aggressive fluid resuscitation [27,28]. Marked changes in both the macro- and microcirculation are believed to be responsible for the deterioration from sepsis to septic shock and the consequent organ dysfunction, organ failure, and death [29–32]. Changes in the microcirculation include a decreased microvascular density and perfusion, as well as increased capillary flow heterogeneity [29,30,33]. Studies have found that microcirculatory changes often precede macrocirculatory changes in humans with sepsis; improvement in microcirculatory derangements is associated with improved survival [29,30,33,34]. Early changes in microcirculatory indices were a stronger predictor of outcome than any macrocirculatory variable monitored in humans with sepsis [35].

Microcirculatory derangements in septic patients are likely multifactorial in origin. These factors include hypovolemia, endothelial cell dysfunction secondary to adhesion molecule expression, increased adhesion of white blood cells, endothelial glycocalyx degradation, uncoupling of connexin, increased permeability of the vascular barrier, formation and lodging of microthrombi, decreased vasomotor autoregulation and reactivity, alterations in local perfusion pressure and flow, and shunting of oxygen to hyperperfused capillary beds [36].

Chapter 6 ◆ The Microcirculation and Fluid Therapy

Based on both experimental and clinical studies, sublingual microcirculatory derangements correlate with microcirculatory changes in other organs such as the intestines and kidneys [37–39]. Changes in the microcirculation in healthy, anesthetized dogs correlate with macrocirculatory measurements of perfusion, although dogs with hemorrhagic shock do not maintain this hemodynamic coherence [40–42]. The correlation in septic dogs has not yet been studied.

Sepsis-induced degradation of the glycocalyx allows plasma proteins and fluid to move across the vascular wall and into the interstitium [43–44]. Damage to the glycocalyx is the result of inflammation and increased circulating "sheddases" (e.g., metalloproteinases, heparinase, and hyaluronidase), which are activated by reactive oxygen species and proinflammatory cytokines [46]. Rodent sepsis studies have elucidated how the endothelial glycocalyx peels away from the endothelial surface and forms spherical bodies that are visible at the injured site [46]. Clinical studies in humans with sepsis have found a decrease in the thickness of the endothelial surface layer that correlated with the severity of critical illness. However, an association between this thickness and microcirculatory imaging parameters such as flow index and the proportion of perfused vessels has not been demonstrated [47].

Monitoring of the microcirculation vs. macrocirculation

There is evidence in the human literature that goal-directed therapy targeting normalization of macrocirculatory parameters may not lead to better outcomes [48–50]. This is likely because the heterogeneity of microcirculatory flow can lead to hypoxic areas, even when treatment successfully normalizes blood flow to organs [30,51]. In an attempt to assess the microcirculation, numerous techniques have been developed and used for diagnostic, prognostic and monitoring purposes. These include laser Doppler, near-infrared spectroscopy, and videomicroscopy [52]. As previously mentioned, macrocirculatory hypoperfusion is linked to microcirculatory derangements; however, microcirculatory dysfunction can occur despite normal macrocirculatory indices. This loss of hemodynamic coherence may result in cryptic shock with hyperlactatemia and acidemia despite adequate perfusion parameters [53]. Both clinical and experimental research has found that normalization of cardiovascular parameters in shock patients may not indicate similar improvements in microcirculatory perfusion [30,33,35,54,55]. Four possible mechanisms that might explain this discrepancy include:

1. Heterogenous effects of inflammatory cytokines on the microcirculation
2. Intravenous fluid administration and subsequent hemodilution

Chapter 6 ◆ The Microcirculation and Fluid Therapy

3. Vasoconstriction of the microcirculation or tamponade from endogenous/exogenous vasopressors and/or increased venous pressure
4. Edematous interstitium from damaged endothelium and glycocalyx [56]

Direct assessment of microcirculatory flow might therefore be a superior monitoring tool for determining the presence of microcirculatory derangements, as well as response to fluid resuscitation.

The use of videomicroscopy techniques such as sidestream dark field (SDF) and incident dark field (IDF) microscopy enable direct imaging of the microcirculation and subsequent determination of vessel density and flow quality [57]. These two technologies require the use of a handheld device that emits green light (530 nm) onto the mucosa of interest; the light is absorbed by the hemoglobin of RBCs in the capillary bed of the tissue. The illuminated RBCs show up as a dark density flowing through the microcirculation, resulting in a real-time magnified video with resolution to allow detection of true capillaries (Figure 6.2). Subsequent analysis of the videos created then generates parameters that reflect the quality and quantity of microcirculatory flow, including total vessel density (TVD), proportion of perfused vessels (PPV), perfused vessel density (PVD), and microvascular flow index (MFI). A standardized approach to microvascular analysis has been published in the human field and provides consensus criteria for the acquisition and analysis of microcirculatory images [58].

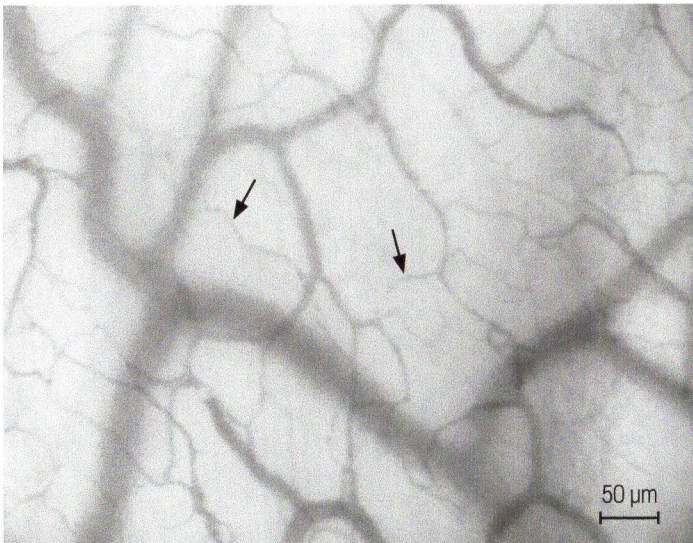

Figure 6.2
Image of microcirculation in a healthy dog using a sidestream dark-field microscopy. Not the plethora of capillaries where only a single cell is able to move through at a time (arrows).

Chapter 6 ◆ The Microcirculation and Fluid Therapy

Direct microvascular imaging has been explored for two decades in human medicine and within the past decade in clinical veterinary medicine [40–41]. However, this technique has not become a standard monitoring tool for the assessment of response to fluid therapy, likely due to the limitations of these technologies. The videomicroscope is expensive, not widely available, and requires the use of thin, mucosal surfaces that are free of pigmentation due to interference with the light technology used for imaging. Generation of quality diagnostic videos for analysis requires training and practice to avoid insufficient or excessive pressure to maximize focus and flow of blood within the microvasculature [58]. Recent advances in the automation of vascular analysis (thereby avoiding time-consuming manual analysis) have proven beneficial; however, the challenges of accuracy remain in the automated vessel assignment used for these calculations, which may lead to inconsistencies in the results. As a result, despite the potential for microvascular imaging to help clinicians evaluating a patient's response to fluid therapy, further improvements in automated vascular analysis and increased availability of the technology are needed before its use can become routine.

In addition to direct imaging of the microcirculation, compromised endothelial glycocalyx integrity can be assessed by measuring shed glycocalyx components in the plasma or serum (e.g., glycosaminoglycans such as hyaluronan, and proteoglycan ectodomains such as syndecan-1). A variety of diseases can lead to damage of the ESL and shedding of the glycocalyx; increased shedding is associated with poor outcomes [59]. There is ongoing research evaluating potential therapeutic strategies that might stimulate repair of a damaged ESL, including specific fluid therapy prescriptions.

The assessment of circulating biomarkers to determine the presence of glycocalyx damage does have limitations. These include the variable methodology used, potential for other causes of biomarker elevations, since most are not unique to the glycocalyx, and upregulation of certain markers with inflammatory or neoplastic diseases. Further details on glycocalyx biomarkers can be found in Chapter 1.

Evaluation of the ESL has been extensively studied in vivo, ex vivo, and in vitro using various techniques that include transmission electron microscopy [60–62], intravital microscopy [63–64], microparticle image velocimetry [65], confocal laser scanning microscopy or atomic force microscopy [66], two-photon laser scanning microscopy [67], and videomicroscopy using handheld devices and different imaging technologies (i.e., orthogonal polarization spectroscopy, sidestream dark field imaging and incident dark field imaging) [68]. Recently, indirect assessment of the glycocalyx has been developed and studied in humans and small animals using the sidestream dark field microscopic technique in conjunction with specialized, proprietary software that measures the vessel lumen width based on RBC movement within as an indirect assessment of glycocalyx thickness (also known as the perfused boundary region or PBR) [69–72]. If there is damage to the ESL, RBCs are able to penetrate further towards the endothelium and the PBR increases [73].

Chapter 6 ◆ The Microcirculation and Fluid Therapy

Effects of fluid resuscitation on the microcirculation in trauma and hemorrhagic shock

Optimizing fluid therapy in the patient suffering from trauma or hemorrhage is often challenging, especially when there is ongoing hemorrhage, as well as progressive anemia, hypoproteinemia and coagulopathy (see Chapter 5). The preferential use of blood products over crystalloids or colloids is commonly recommended in human medicine [74], but the limited natural resources in veterinary medicine frequently result in more frequent use of crystalloids or possibly synthetic colloids. Rodent experimental hemorrhagic shock studies have found that the use of balanced crystalloids, fresh frozen plasma, or concentrated albumin to restore the ESL to be better than normal saline [75–76]. However, results are not consistent, and the use of albumin or fresh frozen plasma has been shown to be more protective than synthetic colloids in a majority of research studies [77]. Additional factors to consider include the rate and volume of administration, but definitive guidelines are lacking. Aggressive fluid administration may exacerbate ongoing hemorrhage, worsen coagulopathy, and injure the endothelial glycocalyx [78–79]. Microcirculatory changes in response to the various fluid types and rates of administration are an area of continued research. As stated above, it is important to recall that improvement of macrovascular parameters does not always correlate with normalization of microvascular perfusion.

How fluid therapy affects the microvasculature in patients with hemorrhagic shock has been the subject of many experimental and preclinical studies. One of the largest systematic reviews of this topic examined 71 articles between 1990 and 2015 and included the use of blood products, hemoglobin-based oxygen carriers, crystalloids and colloids for the management of hemorrhagic shock [80]. The review found that improvements in the microcirculation occurred more commonly with solutions containing hemoglobin vs. those without, fluids that were hyperoncotic vs. those that were not, and fluids that were hyperviscous vs. those that were not [80]. A comparison of hydroxyethyl starch (HES) and saline in an experimental sheep model revealed that saline only improved macrovascular parameters, while HES resulted in better hemodynamic coherence [81]. Despite this, continued concerns about the adverse effects of synthetic colloids on kidney function significantly limit their clinical use in both human and veterinary medicine. It remains unclear whether the use of a dose-restricted, acute volume expansion with synthetic colloids carries a similar risk. In humans suffering from hemorrhagic shock, persistent microcirculatory derangements following resuscitative fluid therapy were more predictive of the development of multiple organ dysfunction syndrome than more commonly studied parameters, such as blood pressure and blood lactate, regardless of the fluid type administered [82].

Chapter 6 ◆ The Microcirculation and Fluid Therapy

Whether or not blood transfusion administration restores microvascular perfusion in patients with hemorrhagic shock is an area of great interest. Packed RBCs were shown to improve microvascular parameters in trauma patients that presented with abnormal values, but there was no change, or even a reduction, in patients that had normal values prior to treatment [83]. A separate pilot study found that although there were no changes in macrovascular parameters or hemoglobin concentrations following an RBC transfusion in human patients with hemorrhagic shock, microvascular perfusion indices did improve significantly [84]. It may be important to take into consideration the duration of blood product storage prior to administration; aged RBC units may have more free hemoglobin, which has been found to scavenge NO and subsequently worsen microvascular blood flow [85]. The use of plasma as a resuscitation fluid in trauma patients is under investigation. Preliminary data suggests that plasma therapy may play an important role in ameliorating immunomodulatory dysfunction and trauma-induced endotheliopathy [86].

Effects of fluid resuscitation on the microcirculation in sepsis

For decades, fluid therapy has been a cornerstone of sepsis treatment. However, the effects of intravenous fluids on microvascular perfusion depend on multiple factors, including the timing and amount of administration, as well as the constituents of the fluids. If fluids are given early to septic patients, microcirculatory parameters improve, but this effect is not seen with fluid administration in the later stages of sepsis [87]. There is some evidence suggesting that bolus fluid therapy worsened survival in people with sepsis [88,89]. Although there was an increase in mean arterial blood pressure, cardiac index, and sublingual microcirculatory RBC velocity following a fluid challenge in humans with abdominal sepsis, intestinal microcirculatory indices were unchanged following administration [90]. Fluids may even contribute to septic endothelial dysfunction and glycocalyx damage, although further research is required [91]. Overall fluid balance in septic patients appears to be of utmost importance; a positive fluid balance is commonly associated with a worse outcome [92–97]. The administration of intravenous crystalloid and colloid fluids was shown to promote endothelial glycocalyx degradation in endotoxemic sheep [98] and humans with sepsis [91,99]. Potential reasons for these findings include:
1. Acute stretching of the vessel wall in the presence of inflammatory mediators could stimulate endothelial expression of glycocalyx-shedding matrix metalloproteinase [100].

Chapter 6 ◆ The Microcirculation and Fluid Therapy

2. An increase in cathepsin L activation (an enzyme that may be involved in post-translational activation of endothelial heparinase) following oscillatory shear stress [101].
3. Triggering of neutrophil-elastase glycocalyx destruction secondary to direct activation of circulating leukocytes [102–104].
4. Increased atrial natriuretic peptide release, which may induce glycocalyx damage [27,105–106].

The type of fluid administered also affects the glycocalyx in septic patients. Both laboratory and clinical data have shown that balanced crystalloids, albumin, fresh frozen plasma, and synthetic colloids may be less injurious than isotonic saline [107–109]. Albumin administration may preserve the glycocalyx along with other benefits when compared to isotonic crystalloids in experimental studies [110–111]; however, research evaluating the glycocalyx following albumin therapy in septic patients is not yet available. Concentrated albumin products enhance the delivery of erythrocyte-derived sphingosine-1-phosphate to the endothelium, which supports glycocalyx recovery by suppressing metalloproteinase activity [112–114]. The use of individualized medicine whereby fluid therapy is determined based on admission markers of endothelial glycocalyx damage might prevent the negative consequences of fluid administration in patients that are prone to vascular endothelial leak syndromes and subsequent organ dysfunction [114].

Conclusion

Coherence between the macro- and microcirculation is often lacking in humans and animals in shock states due to hemorrhage or sepsis. Traditional monitoring strategies may not readily detect microvascular changes in critically ill patients. Intravenous fluid resuscitation plans should consider macrocirculatory upstream parameters (such as systemic arterial blood pressure) as well as downstream measures (such as blood lactate and/or microcirculatory assessments) when monitoring response to treatment. An exciting path for future research might focus on the use of different fluid therapy prescription types, rates, amounts, and goals and their effects on the macro- and microcirculation/endothelial surface layer in various disease states. How these findings affect patient outcome could greatly affect the way clinicians administer fluid resuscitation in the future.

Chapter 6 ◆ The Microcirculation and Fluid Therapy

References

[1] Boulpaep E. The Microcirculation. In: Boron WF, Boulpaep EL (eds.). *Medical Physiology*, 1st ed. Philadelphia: Saunders Elsevier; 2019. pp 463–482.

[2] Sieve I, Münster-Kühnel AK, Hilfiker-Kleiner D. Regulation and function of endothelial glycocalyx layer in vascular diseases. *Vascul Pharmacol*. 2018;100:26–33.

[3] Reines BP, Ninham BW. Structure and function of the endothelial surface layer: unraveling the nanoarchitecture of biological surfaces. *Quarterly Reviews of Biophysics*. 2019;52:e13.

[4] Iba T, Levy JH. Derangement of the endothelial glycocalyx in sepsis. *J Thromb Haemost*. 2019;17(2):283–294.

[5] Weinbaum S, Tarbell JM, Damiano ER. The structure and function of the endothelial glycocalyx layer. *Annu Rev Biomed Eng*. 2007;9:121–167.

[6] Alphonsus CS, Rodseth RN. The endothelial glycocalyx: a review of the vascular barrier. *Anaesthesia*. 2014;69:777–784.

[7] Sieve I, Münster-Kühnel AK, Hilfker-Kleiner D. Regulation and function of endothelial glycocalyx layer in vascular diseases. *Vascul Pharmacol*. 2018;100:26–33.

[8] Becker BF, Chappell D, Jacob M. Endothelial glycocalyx and coronary vascular permeability: the fringe beneft. *Basic Res Cardiol*. 2010;105:687–701.

[9] Esko JD, Kimata K, Lindahl U. Chapter 16. Proteoglycans and sulfated glycosaminoglycans. In: Varki A, Cummings RD, Esko JD et al. (eds). *Essentials of Glycobiology*. Cold Spring Harbor: Cold Spring Harbor Laboratory Press; 2009.

[10] Broekhuizen LN, Mooij HL, Kastelein JJ et al. Endothelial glycocalyx as potential diagnostic and therapeutic target in cardiovascular disease. *Curr Opin Lipidol*. 2009;20:57–62.

[11] Reitsma S, Slaaf DW, Vink H, Nieuwdorp M. The endothelial glycocalyx: composition, functions, and visualization. *Pflug Arch*. 2007;454:345–359.

[12] Woodcock TE, Woodcock TM. Revised Starling equation and the glycocalyx model of transvascular fluid exchange: An improved paradigm for prescribing intravenous fluid therapy. *Br J Anaesth*. 2012; 3:384–394.

[13] Guyton A. Nervous Regulation of the Circulation, and Rapid Control of Arterial Pressure. In: Hall JE (ed.). *Textbook of Medical Physiology*, 13th ed. Philadelphia: Elsevier Inc.; 2016 pp 215–226.

[14] Dinnar U. Metabolic and Mechanical Control of the Microcirculation. In: S. Sideman S, Beyar R (eds.). *Interactive Phenomena in the Cardiac System*. New York: Plenum Press; 2019. pp 243–254.

[15] Guyton A. Dominant Role of the Kidney in Long-Term Regulation of Arterial Pressure and in Hypertension: The Integrated System for Pressure Control. In: Hall JE (ed.). *Textbook of Medical Physiology*, 13th ed. Philadelphia: Elsevier Inc.; 2016. pp 227–244.

[16] Ganong W. Cardiovascular Regulatory Mechanisms. In: Barrett KE, Barman SM, Brooks HL, Yuan J (eds.). *Review of Medical Physiology*, 26th ed. New York: Lange-McGraw-Hill; 2019. pp. 575–588

Chapter 6 ◆ The Microcirculation and Fluid Therapy

[17] Segal S. Regulation of Blood Flow in the Microcirculation. *Microcirculation* 2005;12:33–45.

[18] Cabrales P, Intaglietta M, Tsai AG. Increase plasma viscosity sustains microcirculation after resuscitation from hemorrhagic shock and continuous bleeding. *Shock*. 2005;23(6):549–555.

[19] Dinenno FA. Skeletal muscle vasodilation during systemic hypoxia in humans. *J Appl Physiol*. 2016;120(2):216–225.

[20] Zakaria R, Tsakadze NL, Garrison RN. Hypertonic saline resuscitation improves intestinal microcirculation in a rat model of hemorrhagic shock. *Surgery*. 2006;140:579–587.

[21] Szabo C, Thiemermann C. Invited opinion: role of nitric oxide in hemorrhagic, traumatic, and anaphylactic shock and thermal injury. *Shock*. 1994;2:145–155.

[22] Szopinski J, Kusza K, Semionow M. Microcirculatory responses to hypovolemic shock. *J Trauma*. 2011; 71:1779–1788.

[23] Tachon G, Harrois A, Tanaka S et al. Microcirculatory alterations in traumatic hemorrhagic shock. *Crit Care Med*. 2014;42(6):1433–1441.

[24] Kozar RA, Peng Z, Zhang R et al. Plasma restoration of endothelial glycocalyx in a rodent model of hemorrhagic shock. *Anesth Analg*. 2011;112:1289–1295.

[25] Torres Filho I, Torres LN, Sondeen JL et al. In vivo evaluation of venular glycocalyx during hemorrhagic shock in rats using intravital microscopy. *Microvasc Res*. 2013;85:128–133.

[26] Guerci P, Ergin B, Uz Z et al. Glycocalyx degradation is independent of vascular barrier permeability increase in nontraumatic hemorrhagic shock in rats. *Anesth Analg*. 2019;129:598–607.

[27] Singer M, Deutschman CS, Seymour CW et al. The Third International Consensus Definitions for Sepsis and Septic Shock (Sepsis-3). *JAMA*. 2016;315(8):801–810.

[28] Rhodes A, Evans LE, Alhazzani W et al. Surviving Sepsis Campaign: International Guidelines for Management of Sepsis and Septic Shock: 2016. *Intensive Care Med*. 2017;43(3):304–377.

[29] De Backer D, Creteur J, Preiser JC et al. Microvascular blood flow is altered in patients with sepsis. *Am J Respir Crit Care Med*. 2002;166(1):98–104.

[30] Edul VS, Enrico C, Laviolle B et al. Quantitative assessment of the microcirculation in healthy volunteers and in patients with septic shock. *Crit Care Med*. 2012;40(5):1443-1448.

[31] Massey MJ, Hou PC, Filbin M et al. Microcirculatory perfusion disturbances in septic shock: results from the ProCESS trial. *Crit Care*. 2018;22(1):308.

[32] Shih CC, Liu CM, Chao A et al. Matched Comparison of Microcirculation Between Healthy Volunteers and Patients with Sepsis. *Asian J Anesthesiol*. 2018;56(1):14–22.

[33] Trzeciak S, Dellinger RP, Parrillo JE et al. Early microcirculatory perfusion derangements in patients with severe sepsis and septic shock: Relationship to hemodynamics, oxygen transport, and survival. *Annals of Emergency Medicine*. 2007;49(1):88-98.e2.

Chapter 6 ◆ The Microcirculation and Fluid Therapy

[34] Hernandez G, Boerma EC, Dubin A et al. Severe abnormalities in microvascular perfused vessel density are associated to organ dysfunctions and mortality and can be predicted by hyperlactatemia and norepinephrine requirements in septic shock patients. *J Crit Care*. 2013;28(4):538.e9-14.

[35] De Backer D, Ortiz JA, Salgado D. Coupling microcirculation to systemic hemodynamics. *Curr Opin Crit Care*. 2010;16(3):250–254.

[36] De Backer D, Orbegozo Cortes D, Donadello K, Vincent JL. Pathophysiology of microcirculatory dysfunction and the pathogenesis of septic shock. *Virulence*. 2014;5(1):73–79.

[37] Verdant CL, De Backer D, Bruhn A et al. Evaluation of sublingual and gut mucosal microcirculation in sepsis: a quantitative analysis. *Crit Care Med*. 2009;37(11):2875–2881.

[38] Boerma EC, van der Voort PHJ, Spronk PE, Ince C. Relationship between sublingual and intestinal microcirculatory perfusion in patients with abdominal sepsis. *Crit Care Med*. 2007;35(4):1055–1060.

[39] Lima A, van Rooij T, Ergin B et al. Dynamic Contrast-Enhanced Ultrasound Identifies Microcirculatory Alterations in Sepsis-Induced Acute Kidney Injury. *Crit Care Med*. 2018;46(8):1284–1292.

[40] Silverstein DC, Pruett-Saratan A, Drobatz KJ. Measurements of microvascular perfusion in healthy anesthetized dogs using orthogonal polarization spectral imaging. *J Vet Emerg Crit Care*. 2009;19(6):579–587.

[41] Peruski AM, Cooper ES. Assessment of microcirculatory changes by use of sidestream dark field microscopy during hemorrhagic shock in dogs. *Am J Vet Res*. 2011;72(4):438–445.

[42] An X, Zhang H, Sun Y, Ma X. The microcirculatory failure could not weaken the increase of systematic oxygen extraction rate in septic shock: An observational study in canine models. *Clin Hemorheol Microcirc*. 2016;63(3):267–279.

[43] Chelazzi C, Villa G, Mancinelli P et al. Glycocalyx and sepsis-induced alterations in vascular permeability. *Crit Care*. 2015;19:26.

[44] Fleck A, Hawker F, Wallace PI et al. Increased vascular permeability: a major cause of hypoalbuminaemia in disease and injury. *Lancet*. 1985;325:781–784.

[45] Uchimido R, Schmidt EP, Shapiro NI. The glycocalyx: a novel diagnostic and therapeutic target in sepsis. *Crit Care*. 2019;23(1):16.

[46] Inagawa R, Okada H, Takemura G et al. Ultrastructural alteration of pulmonary capillary endothelial glycocalyx during endotoxemia. *Chest*. 2018 Aug;154(2):317–325.

[47] Rovas A, Seidel LM, Vink H et al. Association of sublingual microcirculation parameters and endothelial glycocalyx dimensions in resuscitated sepsis. *Crit Care*. 2019;23(1):260.

[48] ARISE Investigators, NZICS Clinical Trials Group, Peake SL et al. Goal-directed resuscitation for patients with early septic shock. *N Engl J Med*. 2014;371(16):1496–1506.

[49] PRISM Investigators, Rowan KM, Angus DC et al. Early, Goal-Directed Therapy for Septic Shock — A Patient-Level Meta-Analysis. *N Engl J Med*. 2017;376(23):2223–2234.

[50] Pro CI, Yealy DM, Kellum JA et al. A randomized trial of protocol-based care for early septic shock. *N Engl J Med*. 2014;370(18):1683–1693.

Chapter 6 ◆ The Microcirculation and Fluid Therapy

[51] Ince C, Mik EG. Microcirculatory and mitochondrial hypoxia in sepsis, shock, and resuscitation. *J Appl Physiol*. 2016;120(2):226–235.

[52] De Backer D, Durand A. Monitoring the microcirculation in critically ill patients. *Best Pract Res Clin Anaesthesiol*. 2014;28(4):441–451.

[53] Ranzani OT, Monteiro MB, Ferreira EM et al. Reclassifying the spectrum of septic patients using lactate: severe sepsis, cryptic shock, vasoplegic shock and dysoxic shock. *Rev Bras Ter Intensiva*. 2013;25(4):270–278.

[54] De Backer D, Donadello K, Sakr Y et al. Microcirculatory alterations in patients with severe sepsis: impact of time of assessment and relationship with outcome. *Crit Care Med*. 2013;41(3):791–799.

[55] Tachon G, Harrois A, Tanaka S et al. Microcirculatory alterations in traumatic hemorrhagic shock. *Crit Care Med*. 2014;42(6):1433–1441.

[56] Kara A, Akin S, Ince C. Monitoring microcirculation in critical illness. *Curr Opin Crit Care*. 2016;22(5):444–452.

[57] Ocak I, Kara A, Ince C. Monitoring microcirculation. *Best Pract Res Clin Anaesthesiol*. 2016;30(4):407–418.

[58] Ince C, Boerma EC, Cecconi M et al. Second consensus on the assessment of sublingual microcirculation in critically ill patients: results from a task force of the European Society of Intensive Care Medicine. *Intensive Care Med*. 2018;44:281–299.

[59] Ohansson P, Stensballe J, Ostrowski S. Shock induced endotheliopathy (SHINE) in acute critical illness - a unifying pathophysiologic mechanism. *Crit Care*. 2017;21(1):25.

[60] Janczyk P, Hansen S, Bahramsoltani M, Plendl J. The glycocalyx of human, bovine and murine microvascular endothelial cells cultured in vitro. *J Electron Microsc (Tokyo)*. 2010;59: 291–298.

[61] Pries AR, Secomb TW, Gaehtgens P. The endothelial surface layer. *Pflugers Arch*. 2000; 440: 653–666.

[62] Ebong EE, Macaluso FP, Spray D, Tarbell JM. Imaging the endothelial glycocalyx in vitro by rapid freezing/freeze substitution transmission electron microscopy. *Arterioscler Thromb Vasc Biol*. 2011;31:1908–1915.

[63] Gretz JE, Duling BR. Measurement uncertainties associated with the use of bright-field and fluorescence microscopy in the microcirculation. *Microvasc Res*. 1995;49:134–140.

[64] Kataoka H, Ushiyama A, Kawakami H et al. Fluorescent imaging of endothelial glycocalyx layer with wheat germ agglutinin using intravital microscopy. *Microsc Res Tech*. 2016;79:31–37.

[65] Smith ML, Long DS, Damiano ER, Ley K. Near-wall micro-PIV reveals a hydrodynamically relevant endothelial surface layer in venules in vivo. *Biophys J*. 2003;85:637–645.

[66] Reitsma S, Slaaf DW, Vink H, van Zandvoort MAMJ, oude Egbrink M. The endothelial glycocalyx: composition, functions, and visualization. *Pflugers Arch*. 2007;454:345–359.

[67] Megens RT, Reitsma S, Schiffers PH et al. Two-photon microscopy of vital murine elastic and muscular arteries. Combined structural and functional imaging with subcellular resolution. *J Vasc Res*. 2007;44:87–98.

Chapter 6 ◆ The Microcirculation and Fluid Therapy

[68] Ince C, Boerma EC, Cecconi M et al. Second consensus on the assessment of sublingual microcirculation in critically ill patients: results from a task force of the European Society of Intensive Care Medicine. *Intens Care Med*. 2018;44:281–289.

[69] Londono L, Bowen CM, Buckley GJ. Evaluation of the endothelial glycocalyx in healthy anestheized dogs using rapid, patient-side GlycoCheck analysis software. *J Vet Emerg Crit Care*. 2018;28:S7.

[70] Millar KK, Yozova Y, Londono L et al. Evaluation of the endothelial glycocalyx in healthy anesthetized cats using rapid, patient-side glycocheck analysis software. *J Vet Emerg Crit Care*. 2019;29:S11.

[71] Mullen KM, Regier PJ, Londono L et al. Evaluation of jejunal microvasculature of healthy anaesthetized dogs with sidestream dark field video microscopy. *Am J Vet Res*. 2020;81:888–893.

[72] Yozova ID, Londono L, Sano H et al. Assessment of the endothelial glycocalyx after a fluid bolus in healthy anesthetized cats using rapid, patient-side glycocheck analysis software. *J Vet Emerg Crit Care*. 2020;30:S27.

[73] Lee DH, Dane MJ, van den Berg BM et al. NEO study group. Deeper penetration of erythrocytes into the endothelial glycocalyx is associated with impaired microvascular perfusion. *PLoS One*. 2014 May 9;9(5):e96477.

[74] Dutton RP. Management of traumatic haemorrhage--the US perspective. *Anaesthesia*. 2015;70(Suppl 1):108–11, e38.

[75] Torres LN, Chung KK, Salgado CL et al. Low-volume resuscitation with normal saline is associated with microvascular endothelial dysfunction after hemorrhage in rats, compared to colloids and balanced crystalloids. *Crit Care*. 2017;21(1):160.

[76] Ati S, Potter DR, Baimukanova G et al. Modulating the endotheliopathy of trauma: factor concentrate versus fresh frozen plasma. *J Trauma Acute Care Surg*. 2016;80:576–585.

[77] Milford EM, Reade MC Resuscitation Fluid Choices to Preserve the Endothelial Glycocalyx. *Crit Care*. 2019;23(1):77.

[78] Chappell D, Bruegger D, Potzel J, Jacob M. Hypervolemia increases release of atrial natriuretic peptide and shedding of the endothelial glycocalyx. *Crit Care*. 2014;18(5):538.

[79] Tuma M, Canestrini Z, Alwahab Z, Marshall J. Trauma and endothelial glycocalyx: The Microcirculatory Helmet? Shock 2016;46(4):352–357.

[80] Naumann DN, Beaven A, Dretzke J et al. Searching for the optimal fluid to restore microcirculatory flowdynamcis after hemorrhagic shock: A systematic review of pre-clinical studies. *Shock*. 2016;46(6):609–622.

[81] Amemann P, Hessler M, Kampmeier T et al. Resuscitation with hydroxyethyl starch maintais hemodynamic coherence in ovine hemorrhagic shock. *Anesthesiology*. 2020;132:131–139.

[82] Hutchings SD, Naumann DN, Hopkins P et al. Microcirculatory impairment is associated with multiple organ dysfunction following traumatic hemorrhagic shock: The MICROSHOCK study. *Crit Care Med*. 2018;46(9):889–896.

Chapter 6 ◆ The Microcirculation and Fluid Therapy

[83] Weinberg JA, MacLennan PA, Vandromme-Cusick MJ et al. Microvascular response to red blood cell transfusion in trauma patients. *Shock*. 2012;37(3):276–281.

[84] Tanaka S, Escudier E, Hamada S et al. Effect of RBC transfusion on sublingual microcirculation in hemorrhagic shock patients: A pilot study. *Crit Care Med*. 2017;45(2):154–160.

[85] Damiani E, Adrario E, Luchetti MM et al. Plasma free hemoglobin and microcirculatory response to fresh or old blood transfusions in sepsis. *PLoS One*. 2015;10:e0122655.

[86] Gruen DS, Brown JB, Guyette FX et al. Prehospital plasma is associated with distinct biomarker expression following injury. *JCI*. 2020;5(8):e135350.

[87] Ospina-Tascon G, Neves AP, Occhipinti G, Donadello K. Effects of fluids on microvascular perfusion in patients with severe sepsis. *Intensive Care Med*. 2010; 36:949–955.

[88] Maitland K, Kiguli S, Opoka RO et al. Mortality after fluid bolus in African children with severe infection. *N Engl J Med*. 2011;364:2483–2495.

[89] Andrews B, Semler MW, Muchemwa L et al. Effect of an Early Resuscitation Protocol on In-hospital Mortality Among Adults With Sepsis and Hypotension: A Randomized Clinical Trial. *JAMA*. 2017;318:1233–1240.

[90] Edul VS, Ince C, Navarro N et al. Dissociation between sublingual and gut microcirculation in the response to a fluid challenge in postoperative patients with abdominal sepsis. *Ann Intensive Care*. 2014;4:39.

[91] Hippensteel JA, Uchimido R, Tyler PD et al. Intravenous fluid resuscitation is associated with septic endothelial glycocalyx degradation. *Crit Care*. 2019;23:259.

[92] Silversides JA, Major E, Ferguson AJ et al. Conservative fluid management or deresuscitation for patients with sepsis or acute respiratory distress syndrome following the resuscitation phase of critical illness: a systematic review and meta-analysis. *Intensive Care Med*. 2017;43:155–170.

[93] Marik PE, Linde-Zwirble WT, Bittner EA et al. Fluid administration in severe sepsis and septic shock, patterns and outcomes: an analysis of a large national database. *Intensive Care Med*. 2017;43:625–632.

[94] Acheampong A, Vincent JL. A positive fluid balance is an independent prognostic factor in patients with sepsis. *Crit Care*. 2015;19:251.

[95] Boyd JH, Forbes J, Nakada TA et al. Fluid resuscitation in septic shock: a positive fluid balance and elevated central venous pressure are associated with increased mortality. *Crit Care Med*. 2011;39:259–265.

[96] Sadaka F, Juarez M, Naydenov S, O'Brien J. Fluid resuscitation in septic shock: the effect of increasing fluid balance on mortality. *J Intensive Care Med*. 2014;29:213–217.

[97] Vincent JL, Sakr Y, Sprung CL et al. Sepsis in European intensive care units: results of the SOAP study. *Crit Care Med*. 2006;34:344–353.

[98] Byrne L, Obonyo NG, Diab SD et al. Unintended Consequences: Fluid Resuscitation Worsens Shock in an Ovine Model of Endotoxemia. *Am J Respir Crit Care Med*. 2018;198:1043–1054.

Chapter 6 ◆ The Microcirculation and Fluid Therapy

[99] Chappell D, Bruegger D, Potzel J et al. Hypervolemia increases release of atrial natriuretic peptide and shedding of the endothelial glycocalyx. *Critical Care*. 2014;18:538.

[100] Kang H, Duran CL, Abbey CA et al. Fluid shear stress promotes proprotein convertase-dependent activation of MT1-MMP. *Biochem Biophys Res Commun*. 2015;460:596–602.

[101] Platt MO, Ankeny RF, Jo H. Laminar shear stress inhibits cathepsin L activity in endothelial cells. *Arterioscler Thromb Vasc Biol*. 2006;26:1784–1790.

[102] van Haren FM, Sleigh J, Cursons R et al. The effects of hypertonic fluid administration on the gene expression of inflammatory mediators in circulating leucocytes in patients with septic shock: a preliminary study. *Ann Intensive Care*. 2011;1:44.

[103] Rhee P, Wang D, Ruff P et al. Human neutrophil activation and increased adhesion by various resuscitation fluids. *Crit Care Med*. 2000;28:74–78.

[104] Suzuki K, Okada H, Takemura G et al. Neutrophil Elastase Damages the Pulmonary Endothelial Glycocalyx in Lipopolysaccharide-Induced Experimental Endotoxemia. *Am J Pathol*. 2019;189:1526–1535.

[105] Jacob M, Saller T, Chappell D et al. Physiological levels of A-, B- and C-type natriuretic peptide shed the endothelial glycocalyx and enhance vascular permeability. *Basic Res Cardiol*. 2013;108:347.

[106] Bruegger D, Jacob M, Rehm M et al. Atrial natriuretic peptide induces shedding of endothelial glycocalyx in coronary vascular bed of guinea pig hearts. *Am J Physiol Heart Circ Physiol*. 2005;289:H1993–1999.

[107] Semler MW, Self WH, Wanderer JP et al. Balanced crystalloids versus saline in critically ill adults. *N Engl J Med*. 2018;378(9):829–839.

[108] Finfer S, McEvoy S, Bellomo R et al. Impact of albumin compared to saline on organ function and mortality of patients with severe sepsis. *Intensive Care Med*. 2011;37:86–96.

[109] Müller RB, Ostrowski SR, Haase N et al. Markers of endothelial damage and coagulation impairment in patients with severe sepsis resuscitated with hydroxyethyl starch 130/0.42 vs Ringer acetate. *J Crit Care*. 2016;32:16–20.

[110] Aldecoa C, Llau JV, Nuvials X, Artigas A. Role of albumin in the preservation of endothelial glycocalyx integrity and the microcirculation: a review. *Ann Intensive Care*. 2020; 10:85.

[111] Bansch P, Statkevicius S, Bentzer P. Plasma volume expansion with 5% albumin compared to Ringer's acetate during normal and increased microvascular permeability in the rat. *Anesthesiology*. 2014; 121:817–824.

[112] Adamson RH, Clark JF, Radeva M et al. Albumin modulates S1P delivery from red blood cells in perfused microvessels: mechanism of the protein effect. *Am J Physiol Heart Circ Physiol*. 2014;306:H1011–1017.

[113] Zeng Y, Adamson RH, Curry FRE, Tarbell JM. Sphingosine-1-phosphate protects endothelial glycocalyx by inhibiting syndecan-1 shedding. *Am J Physiol Heart Circ Physiol*. 2014;306:H363–372.

[114] Wu X, Hu Z, Yuan H et al. Fluid Resuscitation and Markers of Glycocalyx Degradation in Severe Sepsis. *Open Med (Wars)*. 2017;12:409–416.

Clinical Case

Microcirculatory changes in a dog with sepsis secondary to bite wounds

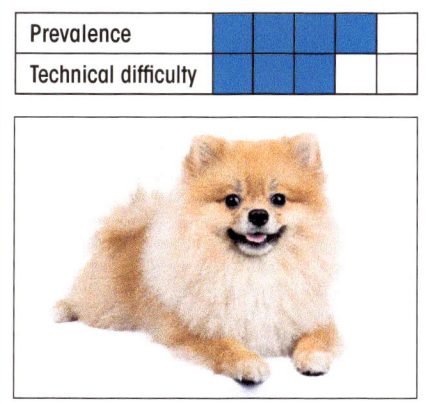

Signalment	
Name	Ginger
Species	canine
Breed	Pomeranian
Sex	male
Age	5 years

History

A 5-year-old male castrated Pomeranian (8 kg) was presented to the emergency clinic 2 days after a fight with the neighbor's Rottweiler. The Pomeranian appeared fine, although shaken, to the owners following the altercation, but had been displaying progressive lethargy and inappetence over the last 48 hours. On the morning of the day of presentation, the dog had vomited bile several times and had been sleeping a lot, which was unusual for him. He also had not eaten breakfast and had passed some soft, tan stool.

Physical examination and initial diagnostics

The dog was mentally dull, estimated 8% dehydrated, and his mucous membranes were bright red with a capillary refill time (CRT) of <1 second. The feet were warm to the touch, femoral pulses were bounding and synchronous with the heartbeat, his heart rate was 178 bpm with no murmurs or arrhythmias, his respiratory rate was 36 bpm, breath sounds were clear in all lungs fields, and his rectal temperature was 39.7 °C. Penetrating bite wounds were discovered over the tail base after clipping the area; purulent material was easily expressed. The skin appeared discolored

Chapter 6 ♦ The Microcirculation and Fluid Therapy

(purple/black) surrounding the puncture wounds and the area measured approximately 8 cm x 5 cm.
Doppler blood pressure: 100 mmHg
SpO_2: 96%
Electrocardiogram: sinus tachycardia
An intravenous catheter was placed in the right cephalic vein and a venous blood gas was obtained, with the following results:

- pH: 7.04;
- pCO_2: 29.3 mmHg;
- pO_2: 27 mmHg;
- Na: 149.1 mmol/L;
- K: 3.23 mmol/L;
- Cl: 113.8 mmol/L;
- Glu: 8.3 mmol/L;
- Lactate: 4.7 mmol/L;
- BE: -18.0 mmol/L;
- $HCO3^-$: 12.2 mmol/L;
- PCV: 46%;
- TP: 78 g/L.

The patient appeared adequately perfused based on the physical examination and blood pressure, but the tachycardia suggested either pain, compensated shock, or systemic inflammation, or a combination of these etiologies (other possibilities do exist as well). The venous blood gas showed a primary metabolic acidosis with respiratory compensation. The increased lactate, decreased base excess, and decreased bicarbonate support a lactic acidosis.

Focused assesment with sonography for trauma of the thorax and abdomen (TFAST and AFAST) were negative (no free fluid or other abnormalities). The left atrium to aorta ratio was 1:1. Chest radiographs were performed and interpreted as unremarkable.

Treatment

Treatment was initiated and included three 10 mL/kg boluses of PlasmaLyte, each over 15–20 minutes. Methadone (0.1 mg/kg IV) and maropitant (1 mg/kg IV) were also administered, and the patient's heart rate following these treatments was 130 bpm, his respiratory rate 28 bpm, his rectal temperature 39.1 °C, and his Doppler blood pressure 120 mmHg. Antimicrobial therapy was initiated using ampicillin (22 mg/kg IV) and enrofloxacin (15 mg/kg IV).

The dog was anesthetized for exploration of the wound. An arterial catheter was placed for direct blood pressure monitoring. A large abscess (8 cm ×12 cm) was identified and drained, flushed, and debrided to remove necrotic skin/subcutaneous tissues. The wound was left open with a wet to dry bandage, which was changed 1-2 times per day as needed. While under general anesthesia, the dog's heart rate was 128 bpm, his respiratory rate 14 bpm and his esophageal temperature 37.8 °C. His mucous membranes were still bright pink with a rapid CRT, and his direct arterial blood pressure was 110/30 with a mean of 58 mmHg. A videomicroscope was used to evaluate the microcirculatory parameters using the vessels in the buccal mucosa. Interpretation was consistent with a decrease in the number of capillaries (see picture below), a decrease in perfusion indices, and a decrease in the microcirculatory flow index. Presumably, cytokines such as NO were causing heterogenous redistribution of blood flow with vasodilation of some capillary beds, but vasoconstriction of others. This created the bright mucous membranes with brisk CRT as well as the bounding pulses (due to a decrease in the diastolic blood pressure while systolic pressure was borderline normal). Although there is no known treatment for microcirculatory derangements, treatment of the underlying inflammatory stimulus and restoration of adequate intravascular volume and albumin are necessary. In this case, removal of the inflammatory stimulus included surgery, debridement, and frequent bandage changes to continue gentle debridement and encourage granulation tissue. Intravenous, broad-spectrum, bactericidal antimicrobial therapy was continued pending aerobic and anaerobic cultures and susceptibility results.

The wound was severely effusive with exudative secretions for 4 hours following surgery and required bandage changes every 8-12 hours due to strike-through of the bandage. The PCV/TP was 33/34 g/L on day 1 postoperatively. The albumin concentration at that time was 14 g/L and the coagulation times were normal. Due to the increased fluid losses from the wound, requirement for high rates of intravenous crystalloids to maintain hydration and intravascular volume, and continued inappetence of the dog, a continuous infusion of cryopoor plasma was initiated at 1.5 mL/kg/hour and continued for 36 hours. This fluid was chosen to decrease the

Chapter 6 ♦ The Microcirculation and Fluid Therapy

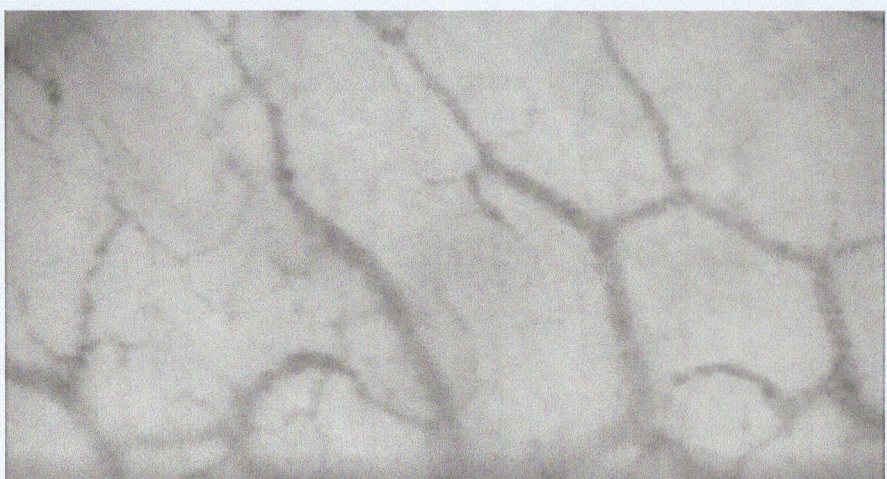

isotonic crystalloid rate to 1 mL/kg/hour while providing a natural source of albumin to prevent a further decrease in the serum albumin concentration and help maintain endothelial integrity.

The dog's clinical signs of sepsis improved, the mucous membranes appeared more normal on day 3 after wound exploration, and the blood pressure and temperature normalized. The dog started eating voluntarily on day 4 post-surgery. Organisms identified from the wound included *Pasteurella canis* and *Neisseria weaveri*. Both were susceptible to amoxicillin–clavulanic acid, so the dog was switched to oral therapy as indicated.

Discharge and follow-up

On day 5 after the initial surgery and debridement, the dog was anesthetized for wound closure. Repeat microcirculatory analysis was performed while the dog was under general anesthesia. There was marked improvement in the microcirculatory capillary numbers, perfusion indices, and microcirculatory flow index, as would be expected based on the clinical improvement in the dog's disease process. The dog was discharged on day 6 and continued his recovery at home. He was prescribed gabapentin for pain and 5 additional days of ampicillin–clavulanic acid. He was doing well at his follow-up examination 2 weeks after discharge.

Subject Index

A

Acid–base balance 142
  chemical species involved 33, 47
  metabolic component 35
Acid–base disorders 31–68
  biological behavior of various components 50
  chemical species involved 34
  complex 34
  correction 55
  diseases associated 40
  interpretation 36
  mixed 34, 39, 40
  nontraditional approach 50
  possible 55
Acid–base disturbance
  chemical species involved 48
  examples 39
  possible 51
  separate primary 38
Acidemia 198
  mild 123
  severe SID 123
Acidosis 33
  lactic 43
  metabolic 43
  paradoxical 34
  respiratory 59
    acute 39
    cronic 39
  weak acid 29
Acute
  bleeding 102
  blood loss 171
  hemorrhage 44, 184
  hypercalcemia 150
  hypercapnia 60
  hypernatremia 141
  hypervolemic 50
  hypoalbuminemia 117
  hyponatremia 137
    treatment 138
  hypotension 108
  lung injury (ALI) 46
  pain 88, 202
  pancreatitis 149
  renal failure 140
  respiratory acidosis 39, 60
  respiratory alkalosis 39
  respiratory distress syndrome (ARDS) 44
  traumatic coagulopathy 188
  tubular necrosis 188
Adenosine triphosphate (ATP) 36, 131, 153, 175
Albumin 115, 184, 185
  canine 185
  human serum (HSA) 184
  iodinated 4
  therapy 209
Aldosterone 142, 174
  secretion 133
Alkalosis 33
  hypoalbuminemic 50
  hypochloremic 50
  hypovolemic 40, 50
  low-protein 50
  metabolic 38, 39, 40
  respiratory 38, 39, 40
    acute 39
    cronic 39
Alveolar–arterial gradient (A–a gradient) 37, 44–45
  measuring 44
Ammonia (NH_3) 130
Angiotensin
  I 133, 172
  II 133, 172, 174
  III 133
  IV 133
  inhibitor 161
Anion gap (AG) 37, 41
  and metabolic acidosis 43
  high 40
  increased 43
  normal 40, 43
  strong 49
Anions 129
  measured 41
  nondiffusible 142
  unmeasured (UAs) 41, 50, 51
Anticonvulsant drugs 149
Aquaporins 134
Arrhythmias 152, 160, 161, 186, 188
  ventricular 144
Atomic force microscopy 206
Atrial fibrillation 160

Subject Index

Autologous blood transfusion 187
Autotransfusion 23, 187

B

Balanced crystalloids 207, 209
Balanced isotonic solutions 56, 62, 109
Base excess (BE) 41
Blood gas analysis
  interpretation of
    compensatory responses 38
  normal values of
    in cats 37
    in dogs 37
    primary disorder 38
Blood gas analyzers 36
Blood pressure (BP) 86
Blood products 182
Blood volume (BV) 5
  assessment of
    CVC (caudal vena cava) diameter 14
    CVCCI (CVC diameter variations) 14
    POCUS (point-of-care ultrasound) 14
  measurement 13
  parameters to evaluate 14
Body fluids 129
  evaluate 14
  output 79
Body temperature 84
Bradycardia 173

C

Calcitonin 148, 152
Calcium 147
  distribution in plasma 148
  hypercalcemia 151
  hypocalcemia 149
Calcium imbalances
  treatment of 150
Calciuresis 152
Canine eclampsia 149
Capillary phenotypes 21
Capillary refill time (CRT) 83
Carbonic acid (H_2CO_3) 130
Cardiac functionality index (CFI) 5
Cardiac output (CO) 5
  evaluation 13
  methods to assess with calibration 6
  parameters to evaluate 14
    bioimpedance 14
    electrical velocimetry 14
    esophageal doppler 14
    transesophageal echocardiography 14
Cardiogenic shock
  consequences and therapy 91
Catecholamines 198, 142
Cations 129
Cellular
  metabolic homeostasis 173
  necrosis 142
Cell wall membrane 130
Central diabetes insipidus 139
Central venous pressure (CVP) 14
Chloremia 156
  alterations in 156
Chloride 156
  hyperchloremia 156
  hypochloremia 157
Chloride imbalances
  treatment of 158
Chronic kidney disease 152
Clinical hemodynamic
  monitoring 15
Coagulopathy 176, 207
Colloid oncotic pressure 18
Colloids 99, 112
  composition of 103
  natural 115
  synthetic 113
Compartmentalization
  of fluids in the body 1
Compensatory shock 172
Confocal laser scanning microscopy 206
Corticosteroid deficiency 151
Crystalloids 99, 106, 109
  composition of 74

D

Daily electrolyte
  in cats 75
  in dogs 75
Daily fluid therapy 77
  calculation of 79

Subject Index

Daily water
  maintenance 75
  requirements 72
Decompensatory shock 173
  early 173
  late 173
Dehydration
  clinical signs of 79
Dextran solutions 113
Dilutional coagulopathy 180
Dog
  dehydrated
    with respiratory alkalosis 27
Doppler ultrasonic method 90

E

Early decompensatory shock 173
Edema 180
Edematous interstitium 205
Electrolyte and acid–base imbalances
        during vomiting 163
Electrolyte disorders 127–168
  calcium 147
  chloride 156
  clinical case 163
  hypercalcemia 151
  hyperchloremia 156
  hyperkalemia 144
  hypermagnesemia 161
  hypernatremia 139
  hypocalcemia 149
  hypochloremia 157
  hypomagnesaemia 159
  hyponatremia 135
  hypophosphatemia 154
  introduction 129
  magnesium 158
  osmosis 130
  phosphorus 153
    imbalances 155
  potassium 142
  sodium 132
End-diastolic volume index (EDVI) 11
Endothelin 198
Esophageal Doppler 13
Evaluation of stroke volume 13
Evidence-based medicine (EBM) 3

Extracellular fluid (ECF) 129
Extrarenal losses 143
Extra vascular lung water (EVLW) 5, 11

F

Fanconi syndrome 154
Fasciculations 149
Feline idiopathic hypercalcemia 151
Fluid compartments 17
  dynamics 4
  extracellular fluid (ECF) 17
  hemodynamics 4
  intracellular fluid (ICF) 17
Fluid kinetics 108
Fluid resuscitation 97
  with colloids 102
  with crystalloids 102
Fluids
  how to administer 69
  when to administer 69–126
Fluid therapy 3
  and antidiuretic hormone 76
  and SID 52
  daily intravenous 71
  fundamentals of 1–30
  goal-directed therapy 98
  indications 4
  in hemorrhagic shock
    albumin 184
    autotransfusion 187
    blood products 182
    fresh frozen plasma transfusion 183
    hemoglobin-based oxygen carriers 186
    hypertonic solutions 181
    isotonic crystalloids 180
    massive transfusion 186
    packed red blood cell transfusion 183
    platelet transfusion 185
    synthetic colloids 182
    whole blood transfusion 183
  objectives 91
  ROSE model 105
  under general anesthesia 77
Fluid volume 73
  and complications 73
  under general anesthesia 77
Fresh frozen plasma transfusion 183

Subject Index

G

Gastroenteritis 121
Gibbs–Donnan effect 130
Global end-diastolic volume (GEDV) 5
Glomerular
  filtration 134
  perfusion 134
Glucagon 142
Glucocorticoids 152
Glycocalyx 19, 198
  biomarkers 206
Glycocalyx model
  clinical consequences 22, 24
Glycolysis 175
Granulomatous meningoencephalitis 135

H

Heart rate
  and cardiac output 81
Heartworm disease 135
Hemodialysis 147
Hemodynamic assessment
  dynamic parameters 87
  static parameters 87
Hemodynamic monitoring 80
Hemodynamic parameters
  dynamic 8
  static 8
Hemodynamic response 13
  monitoring 13
  parameters to evaluate the 8
    hemodynamic support 13
    PI (perfusion index) 13
    PPV (pulse pressure variation) 13
    PVI (pleth variability index) 13
Hemodynamics
  of fluids in the body 1–30
Hemodynamic status
  parameters to evaluate 86
Hemoglobin based oxygen carriers 186
Hemorrhage 171, 172, 174
  control 176
  induced hypotension 173
  moderate normotensive 173
  treatment 176

Hemorrhagic shock 169–194
  and microvascular changes 202
  clinical case 191
  clinical management 179
  compensatory shock 172
  diagnosis 177
    laboratory data 177
    monitoring 177
    shock index 178
    ultrasonography 178
  etiology of 176
  following a ruptured hepatocellular
        carcinoma 191
  fluid therapy in 180
  hypotensive resuscitation 179
  introduction 171
  metabolic sequelae of 175
  pathophysiology of 171
  postresuscitation care 188
    reperfusion injury 188
  trauma-induced coagulopathy 188
  triage 179
Henderson–Hasselbalch equation 35
Hydration 78
Hydrocephalus 135
Hydrochloric acid 130
Hydrostatic pressure 23
Hydroxyapatite 147
Hydroxyethyl starches (HES) 114, 207
Hypercalcemia 151
  clinical signs 152
  treatment 152
Hypercapnia 179, 198
Hypercarbia 172
Hyperchloremia 156
  clinical signs 157
  treatment 157
Hyperkalemia 144
  clinical signs 146
  correction of 145
  treatment 146
Hyperlactatemia 204
Hypermagnesemia 161
Hypernatremia 139
  clinical signs 140
  treatment 141
Hyperosmolality 142
Hyperphosphatemia 153
  clinical signs 154

Subject Index

treatment 154
Hypertonic solutions 111, 181
Hypervitaminosis D 152
Hypervolemia 6
Hypocalcemia 149
  clinical signs 149
  treatment 150
Hypochloremia 157
  treatment 158
Hypokalemia 143
  clinical signs 143
  treatment 144
Hypokalemia correction 145
Hypomagnesemia 159
  clinical signs 160
  diagnosis 160
  etiology 159
  treatment 160
Hypomagnesemia
  and gastrointestinal pathologies 159
  and renal pathologies 160
Hyponatremia 135
  clinical signs 137
  treatment 137
  with hypervolemia 137
  with hypovolemia 136
  with increased plasma osmolality 135
  with normal osmolality 135
  with normovolemia 135
  with reduced plasma osmolality 135
Hypoparathyroidism 151
Hypophosphatemia 154
  clinical signs 155
  treatment 155
Hypoproteinemia 207
Hypotensive resuscitation 179
Hypotonic solutions 73
Hypovolemia 6
Hypovolemic shock 173
Hypoxemia 172, 179
Hypoxia 198

I

Iatrogenic hyperchloremia 156
Increased
  absorption of intestinal calcium 151
  intestinal absorption 154

PTH production 151
Insufficient PTH production 149
Intoxication by ethylene glycol 149
Intracellular fluid (ICF) 129
Intrathoracic total blood volume (ITBV) 5
Intravascular hemolysis 155
Intravital microscopy 206
Invasive blood pressure (IBP)
  measurement
    indications 94
    interpretation 94
    technique 94
Ionization 130
Isotonic crystalloids 180
Isotonic saline solutions 110

J

Jugular vein distension 85

L

Lactatemia
  measurement 96
Late decompensatory shock 173
Left ventricular volume score
    (LVVS) 11
Lithium dilution cardiac output
    (LiDCO) 5
Lithium thermodilution (LiDCO System) 5
Loop of Henle 134

M

Macrocirculatory hypoperfusion 204
Magnesium 158
  hypermagnesemia 161
  hypomagnesemia 159
Magnesium imbalances
  treatment of 161
Malignant neoplasms 151
Massive transfusion 186
Mean arterial pressure (MAP) 90
Measurement of invasive blood
    pressure (IBP) 92

Subject Index

Meningioma 139
Metabolic acidosis 39, 40
  and anion gap 43
  sodium bicarbonate therapy 56
  treatment 56
Metabolic alkalosis 39, 40, 57
  treatment 59
Metatarsal artery 93
Methylprednisolone 161
Microcirculation
  and fluid therapy 195–220
  effects of fluid resuscitation 207
    on the microcirculation in sepsis 208
  microvascular changes with sepsis 203
  microvascular changes with trauma and hemorrhagic shock 202
  microvascular perfusion
    local control 201
  microvascular perfusion
    systemic control 198
  monitoring of the microcirculation vs. macrocirculation 204
  schematic of the 199
  structure and function 197
  vs. macrocirculation 204
Microcirculatory changes and sepsis secondary to bite wounds 217
Microcirculatory derangements 205
Microparticle image velocimetry 206
Microvascular changes
  with sepsis 203
  with trauma and hemorrhagic shock 202
Microvascular imaging 206
Microvascular perfusion 201
Mixed disorders 61
  treatment 62
Mucous membrane color 84
Muscle cramping 149
Muscle tremors 149

N

Neoplasms of the hypothalamus 135
Nephrotic syndrome 157
Noninvasive blood pressure (NIBP) 88
Nonsignificant hypercalcemia 151

Normal blood pressure values
  in cats 89
  in dogs 89
Normotensive resuscitation 180

O

Oncotic pressure
  formula 18
Osmolality 131
Osmoreceptors 132
Osmosis 130
  osmolarity and osmolality 131
Osmotic pressure 16, 132
  formula 18
  of the solute 130
Oxidative phosphorylation 131
Oxygenation
  oxygen parameters 44

P

Packed cell volume (PCV) 177
Packed red blood cell transfusion 183
Pancreatic hormones 142
PaO_2/FiO_2 ratio 45
  clinical interpretation 46
Parameters to evaluate
  cardiac output 14
Paraneoplastic hypocalcemia 149
Parathyroid hormone 147
Perfusion
  clinical parameters 81
pH
  effects of chemical species 36
Phosphorus 153
  hyperphosphatemia 153
  hypophosphatemia 154
  maldistribution of 154
  reduced renal excretion of 154
  phosphorus imbalances 155
PiCCO (pulse contour cardiac output) 5
Plasma–Lyte 111
Plasma osmolarity 132
Platelet transfusion 185
Point-of-care ultrasound (POCUS) 8
Polydipsia 149, 152

Subject Index

Polyuria 149, 152
Potassium disorders 142
  hyperkalemia 144
  hypokalemia 143
Potassium imbalances
  treatment of 145
Potassium supplementation 145
Primary pituitary neoplasia 139
Pseudohypercalcemia 151
Pseudohypochloremia 157
Pseudohypokalemia 143
Psychogenic polydipsia 135
Puerperal eclampsia 149
Pulmonary artery occlusion pressure
      (PAOP) 14
Pulmonary capillary wedge pressure
      (PCWP) 14
Pulse CO System 5
Pulse quality 82

R

Redistributive hypokalemia 143
Reduced renal excretion 151
Renal failure 149
Renal juxtaglomerular cells 172
Renal losses 143
Renin 133
Renin–angiotensin–aldosterone system
      (RAAS) 133, 172
Reperfusion injury 188
Respiratory acidosis 40, 59
  acute 39
  chronic 39
  treatment 60
Respiratory alkalosis 40
  treatment 61
  acute 39
  chronic 39
Ringer's solutions 110
ROSE model 104
Rule of 5 47, 120 47

S

Saline solution 110
Sepsis 149, 208

Shock
  cardiogenic, consequences
      and therapy 91
  distributive, consequences
      and therapy 91
  hypovolemic, consequences
      and therapy 91
Shock index 178
Sodium 132
  hypernatremia 139
  hyponatremia 135
Sodium chloride 131
Sodium hydroxide (NaOH) 130
Solutes 129
Spironolactone 161
Stranguria
  in cat 63
Stroke volume (SV) 5
  parameters to evaluate 14
    bioimpedance 14
    electrical velocimetry 14
    esophageal doppler 14
    transesophageal echocardiography 14
  variation (SVV) 5
Strong ions 54
Strong ion gap (SIG) 55
Strong ion theory (Stewart's approach) 47
Supraventricular tachycardia 160
Syndrome of inappropriate
      antidiuretic hormone secretion
      (SIADH) 135, 157
Synthetic colloids 182
Systemic vascular resistance
      (SVR) 5, 172

T

Tachycardia 160
Tachypnea 173
Thrombocytopenia 155, 176
Thromboxane 198
Total oxygen content (CaO_2) 43
Total vessel density (TVD) 205
Transmission electron microscopy 206
Transvascular filtration 23
Trauma
  and microvascular changes 202

Subject Index

Trauma-induced
   coagulopathy 188
   endotheliopathy 208
Two-photon laser scanning microscopy 206

U

Unbalanced solutions 109
Urethral obstruction
   treatment 67
Urine production 86

V

Vascular smooth muscle tone 200
Vasoconstrictors 200
Vasodilators 200

Vasopressin 132
   release 172
Ventricular
   contractility, 172
   ectopic beats 160
   tachycardia 160
Videomicroscopy techniques 205

W

Water 4
   daily requirements 72
     in cats 75
     in dogs 75
   distribution
     in the body 16
   reabsorption 134
   retention 52
Whole blood transfusion 183